PEDIATRICS, CHILD AND ADOLESCENT HEALTH

ADOLESCENCE IN CURAÇAO

PEDIATRICS, CHILD AND ADOLESCENT HEALTH

JOAV MERRICK - SERIES EDITOR

NATIONAL INSTITUTE OF CHILD HEALTH AND HUMAN DEVELOPMENT,
MINISTRY OF SOCIAL AFFAIRS, JERUSALEM

Adolescence in Curaçao
Soraya Verstraeten, Supa Pengpid, Karl Peltzer and Joav Merrick (Editors)
2020. ISBN: 978-1-53617-522-6 (softcover)
2020. ISBN: 978-1-53617-523-3 (e-book)

Building Youth for the Future: Suicide Prevention Aspects
Hatim A. Omar *and Joav Merrick (Editors)*
2019. ISBN: 978-1-53615-799-4 (Hardcover)
2019. ISBN: 978-1-53616-565-4 (e-book)

Vaccine: Measles and Rubella Vaccination Experience in Zambia
Mazyanga L. Mazaba-Liwewe, Seter Siziya and Joav Merrick (Editors)
2019. ISBN: 978-1-53615-799-4 (Hardcover)
2019. ISBN: 978-1-53615-800-7 (e-book)

The Boko Haram Terror: Adversary to the Wellbeing of Nigerian Kids
Miracle A. Adesina, Kehinde K. Kanmodi and Joav Merrick (Editors)
2019. ISBN: 978-1-53615-443-6 (Softcover)
2019. ISBN: 978-1-53615-444-3 (e-book)

Chronic Disease and Disability: Pediatric Obesity Perspectives
Marisha Agana, Donald E. Greydanus, Manmohan K. Kamboj and Joav Merrick (Editors)
2019. ISBN: 978-1-53615-240-1 (Hardcover)
2019. ISBN: 978-1-53615-241-8 (e-book)

Substance Use Disorders in Adolescents and Young Adults: A Manual for Pediatric and Primary Care Clinicians. Second Edition

Donald E. Greydanus, Gabriel Kaplan, Dilip R. Patel and Joav Merrick (Editors)

2019. ISBN: 978-1-53615-359-0 (Hardcover)

2019. ISBN: 978-1-53615-360-6 (e-book)

Building Youth for the Future: A Path towards Suicide Prevention

Hatim A. Omar and Joav Merrick (Editors)

2018. ISBN: 978-1-53613-768-2 (Hardcover)

2018. ISBN: 978-1-53613-769-9 (e-book)

Soft Skills and Aspirations in Chinese Children and Youth

Daniel T.L. Shek, Janet TY Leung and Joav Merrick (Editors)

2018. ISBN: 978-1-53614-092-7 (Hardcover)

2018. ISBN: 978-1-53614-093-4 (e-book)

Childhood and Adolescence: Tribute to Emanuel Chigier, 1928-2017

Joav Merrick (Editor)

2018. ISBN: 978-1-53613-574-9 (Hardcover)

2018. ISBN: 978-1-53613-574-9 (e-book)

Child Health and Human Development Yearbook 2017

Joav Merrick (Editor)

2018. ISBN: 978-1-53613-628-9 (Hardcover)

2018. ISBN: 978-1-53613-629-6 (e-book)

Child and Adolescent Health Yearbook 2017

Joav Merrick (Editor)

2018. ISBN: 978-1-53613-594-7 (Hardcover)

2018. ISBN: 978-1-53613-595-4 (e-book)

Chronic Disease and Disability: The Pediatric Gastrointestinal Tract

Donald E Greydanus, Orhan Atay, and Joav Merrick (Editors)

2018. ISBN: 978-1-53612-948-9 (Hardcover)

2018. ISBN: 978-1-53612-949-6 (e-book)

Multiple Sclerosis in Children and Adolescents
Hatim Omar and Joshua Chalkley (Editors)
2018. ISBN: 978-1-53612-979-3 (Hardcover)
2018. ISBN: 978-1-53612-980-9 (e-book)

Childhood and Adolescence: Tribute to Emanuel Chigier, 1928-2017
Joav Merrick (Editor)
2018. ISBN: 978-1-53613-574-9 (Softcover)
2018. ISBN: 978-1-53613-575-6 (e-book)

Chronic Disease and Disability: The Pediatric Lung
Donald E Greydanus, Myrtha M Gregoire-Bottex, Kevin W Cates and Joav Merrick (Editors)
2018. ISBN: 978-1-53613-577-0 (Hardcover)
2018. ISBN: 978-1-53613-578-7 (e-book)

Bicycles: Helmet Use of Adolescents at Independent Schools
Ronald Chow, Michael Borean, Drew Hollenberg, Jaclyn Viehweger, Tharani Anpalagan and Anna Rzepka (Editors)
2017. ISBN: 978-1-53612-458-3 (Hardcover)
2017. ISBN: 978-1-53612-459-0 (e-book)

Positive Youth Development: Long Term Effects in a Chinese Program
Daniel TL Shek, Cecilia MS Ma, Janet TY Leung and Joav Merrick (Editors)
2017. ISBN: 978-1-53612-539-9 (Hardcover)
2017. ISBN: 978-1-53612-540-5 (e-book)

Adolescence: Bicycle and Helmet Use of Adolescents and Young Adults
Ronald Chow and Joav Merrick (Editors)
2017. ISBN: 978-1-53612-039-4 (Hardcover)
2017. ISBN: 978-1-53612-060-8 (e-book)

Suicide: A Global View on Suicidal Ideation among Adolescents
Mazyanga L. Mazaba, Seter Siziya and Joav Merrick (Editors)
2017. ISBN: 978-1-53611-788-2 (Hardcover)
2017. ISBN: 978-1-53611-799-8 (e-book)

Children and Youth: Post-Traumatic Stress Disorder and Motor Vehicle Crashes
Donald E. Greydanus, Roger W. Apple, Kathryn White, and Joav Merrick (Editors)
2017. ISBN: 978-1-53611-102-6 (Hardcover)
2017. ISBN: 978-1-53611-255-9 (e-book)

Child and Adolescent Health Yearbook 2016
Joav Merrick (Editor)
2017. ISBN: 978-1-53610-948-1 (Hardcover)
2017. ISBN: 978-1-53610-957-3 (e-book)

Child Health and Human Development Yearbook 2016
Joav Merrick (Editor)
2017. ISBN: 978-1-53610-946-7 (Hardcover)
2017. ISBN: 978-1-53610-958-0 (e-book)

Chronic Disease and Disability: The Pediatric Kidney
Donald E Greydanus, Vimal Master Sankar Raj, and Joav Merrick (Editors)
2016. ISBN: 978-1-63483-793-4 (Hardcover)
2015. ISBN: 978-1-63483-809-2 (e-book)

Child and Adolescent Health Yearbook 2015
Joav Merrick (Editor)
2016. ISBN: 978-1-63484-512-0 (Hardcover)
2016. ISBN: 978-1-63484-543-4 (e-book)

Child Health and Human Development Yearbook 2015
Joav Merrick (Editor)
2016. ISBN: 978-1-63484-513-7 (Hardcover)
2016. ISBN: 978-1-63484-544-1 (e-book)

Pain Management Yearbook 2015
Joav Merrick (Editor)
2016. ISBN: 978-1-63484-515-1 (Hardcover)
2016. ISBN: 978-1-63484-545-8 (e-book)

Children and Childhood: Some International Aspects
Joav Merrick (Editor)
2016. ISBN: 978-1-63484-587-8 (Hardcover)
2016. ISBN: 978-1-63484-594-6 (e-book)

Children and Adolescents: Future Challenges
Daniel TL Shek, Tak Yan Lee, and Joav Merrick (Editors)
2016. ISBN: 978-1-63484-616-5 (Hardcover)
2016. ISBN: 978-1-63484-627-1 (e-book)

Adolescence: Positive Youth Development Programs in Chinese Communities
Daniel TL Shek, Florence KY Wu, Janet TY Leung, and Joav Merrick (Editors)
2016. ISBN: 978-1-63484-044-6 (Hardcover)
2016. ISBN: 978-1-63484-677-6 (e-book)

Sexuality: Some International Aspects
Joav Merrick and Donald E Greydanus (Editors)
2016. ISBN: 978-1-63484-707-0 (Hardcover)
2016. ISBN: 978-1-63484-719-3 (e-book)

Growing Up in the Middle East: The Daily Lives and Well-Being of Israeli and Palestinian Youth
Yossi Harel-Fisch, Ziad Abdeen and Miriam Navot
2016. ISBN: 978-1-63484-746-9 (Hardcover)
2016. ISBN: 978-1-63484-765-0 (e-book)

Chronic Disease and Disability: The Pediatric Heart
Donald E Greydanus, Devika Malhotra and Joav Merrick (Editors)
2016. ISBN: 978-1-63484-828-2 (Hardcover)
2016. ISBN: 978-1-63484-842-8 (e-book)

Diabetes Mellitus: Childhood and Adolescence
Manmohan K Kamboj, Donald E Greydanus and Joav Merrick (Editors)
2016. ISBN: 978-1-53610-095-2 (Hardcover)
2016. ISBN: 978-1-53610-104-1 (e-book)

Chronic Disease and Disability: Abuse and Neglect in Childhood and Adolescence
Donald E Greydanus, Vincent J Palusci and Joav Merrick (Editors)
2016. ISBN: 978-1-53610-129-4 (Hardcover)
2016. ISBN: 978-1-53610-142-3 (e-book)

Clinical Aspects of Psychopharmacology in Childhood and Adolescence, Second Edition
Donald E Greydanus, Joseph L Calles, Jr, Dilip R Patel, Ahsan Nazeer and Joav Merrick (Editors)
2016. ISBN: 978-1-53610-241-3 (Hardcover)
2016. ISBN: 978-1-53610-253-6 (e-book)

Chronic Disease and Disability: The Pediatric Pancreas
Donald E Greydanus, Manmohan K Kamboj and Joav Merrick (Editors)
2016. ISBN: 978-1-53610-055-6 (Hardcover)
2016. ISBN: 978-1-53610-065-5 (e-book)

A Pediatric Resident Pocket Guide: Making the Most of Morning Reports
Arthur N Feinberg
2015. ISBN: 978-1-63482-141-4 (Softcover)
2015. ISBN: 978-1-63482-186-5 (e-book)

Tropical Pediatrics: A Public Health Concern of International Proportions Second Edition
Richard R Roach, Donald E Greydanus, Dilip R Patel and Joav Merrick (Editors)
2015. ISBN: 978-1-63463-381-9 (Hardcover)
2015. ISBN: 978-1-63463-404-5 (e-book)

Child and Adolescent Health Issues (A Tribute to the Pediatrician Donald E Greydanus)
Joav Merrick (Editor)
2015. ISBN: 978-1-63463-574-5 (Hardcover)
2015. ISBN: 978-1-63463-576-9 (e-book)

Child and Adolescent Health Yearbook 2014
Joav Merrick (Editor)
2015. ISBN: 978-1-63482-162-9 (Hardcover)
2015. ISBN: 978-1-63482-206-0 (e-book)

Child Health and Human Development Yearbook 2014
Joav Merrick (Editor)
2015. ISBN: 978-1-63482-163-6 (Hardcover)
2015. ISBN: 978-1-63482-207-7 (e-book)

Behavioral Pediatrics, 4th Edition
Donald E Greydanus, Dilip R Patel, Helen D Pratt, Joseph L Calles Jr, Ahsan Nazeer and Joav Merrick (Editors)
2015. ISBN: 978-1-63483-027-0 (Hardcover)
2015. ISBN: 978-1-63483-052-2 (e-book)

Disability, Chronic Disease and Human Development
Joav Merrick
2015. ISBN: 978-1-63483-029-4 (Hardcover)
2015. ISBN: 978-1-63483-057-7 (e-book)

Caribbean Adolescents: Some Public Health Concerns
Cecilia Hegamin-Younge and Joav Merrick (Editors)
2015. ISBN: 978-1-63483-341-7 (Hardcover)
2015. ISBN: 978-1-63483-343-1 (e-book)

Adolescence and Health: Some International Perspectives
Joav Merrick (Editor)
2015. ISBN: 978-1-63483-791-0 (Hardcover)
2015. ISBN: 978-1-63483-808-5 (e-book)

Youth Suicide Prevention: Everybody's Business
Hatim A Omar (Editor)
2015. ISBN: 978-1-63483-786-6 (Softcover)
2015. ISBN: 978-1-63483-820-7 (e-book)

Human Developmental Research: Experience from Research in Hong Kong
Daniel TL Shek, Cecilia Ma, Yu Lu and Joav Merrick (Editors)
2014. ISBN: 978-1-62808-166-4 (Hardcover)
2013. ISBN: 978-1-62808-167-1 (e-book)

School, Adolescence and Health Issues
Joav Merrick, Ariel Tenenbaum and Hatim A Omar (Editors)
2014. ISBN: 978-1-62948-702-1 (Hardcover)
2014. ISBN: 978-1-62948-707-6 (e-book)

Adolescence and Sexuality: International Perspectives
Joav Merrick, Ariel Tenenbaum and Hatim A Omar (Editors)
2014. ISBN: 978-1-62948-711-3 (Hardcover)
2014. ISBN: 978-1-62948-724-3 (e-book)

Child and Adolescent Health Yearbook 2013
Joav Merrick (Editor)
2014. ISBN: 978-1-63117-658-6 (Hardcover)
2014. ISBN: 978-1-63117-668-5 (e-book)

Adoption: The Search for a New Parenthood
Gary Diamond and Eva Arbel
2014. ISBN: 978-1-63117-710-1 (Hardcover)
2014. ISBN: 978-1-63117-713-2 (e-book)

Adolescence: Places and Spaces
Myra F Taylor, Julie Ann Pooley and Joav Merrick (Editors)
2014. ISBN: 978-1-63117-847-4 (Hardcover)
2014. ISBN: 978-1-63117-850-4 (e-book)

Pain Management Yearbook 2013
Joav Merrick (Editor)
2014. ISBN: 978-1-63117-944-0 (Hardcover)
2014. ISBN: 978-1-63117-959-4 (e-book)

Child Health and Human Development Yearbook 2013
Joav Merrick (Editor)
2014. ISBN: 978-1-63117-939-6 (Hardcover)
2013. ISBN: 978-1-63117-958-7 (e-book)

Born into this World: Health Issues
Donald E Greydanus, Arthur N Feinberg, and Joav Merrick (Editors)
2014. ISBN: 978-1-63321-667-9 (Hardcover)
2014. ISBN: 978-1-63321-669-3 (e-book)

Caring for the Newborn: A Comprehensive Guide for the Clinician
Donald E Greydanus, Arthur N Feinberg and Joav Merrick (Editors)
2014. ISBN: 978-1-63321-760-7 (Hardcover)
2014. ISBN: 978-1-63321-781-2 (e-book)

Environment and Hope: Improving Health, Reducing AIDS and Promoting Food Security in the World
Leslie Rubin and Joav Merrick (Editors)
2014. ISBN: 978-1-63321-772-0 (Hardcover)
2014. ISBN: 978-1-63321-782-9 (e-book)

Pediatric and Adolescent Dermatology: Some Current Issues
Donald E Greydanus, Arthur N Feinberg and Joav Merrick (Editors)
2014. ISBN: 978-1-63321-853-6 (Hardcover)
2014. ISBN: 978-1-63321-863-5 (e-book)

Adolescence and Behavior Issues in a Chinese Context
Daniel TL Shek, Rachel CF Sun, and Joav Merrick (Editors)
2013. ISBN: 978-1-62618-614-9 (Hardcover)
2013. ISBN: 978-1-62618-692-7 (e-book)

Advances in Preterm Infant Research
Jing Sun, Nicholas Buys and Joav Merrick
2013. ISBN: 978-1-62618-696-5 (Hardcover)
2013. ISBN: 978-1-62618-775-7 (e-book)

Child Health and Human Development: Social, Economic and Environmental Factors
Leslie Rubin and Joav Merrick (Editors)
2013. ISBN: 978-1-62948-166-1 (Hardcover)
2013. ISBN: 978-1-62948-169-2 (e-book)

Children, Violence and Bullying: International Perspectives
Joav Merrick, Isack Kandel and Hatim A Omar (Editors)
2013. ISBN: 978-1-62948-342-9 (Hardcover)
2013. ISBN: 978-1-62948-345-0 (e-book)

Chinese Adolescent Development: Economic Disadvantages, Parents and Intrapersonal Development
Daniel TL Shek, Rachel CF Sun and Joav Merrick (Editors)
2013. ISBN: 978-1-62618-622-4 (Hardcover)
2013. ISBN: 978-1-62618-694-1 (e-book)

Chronic Disease and Disability in Childhood
Joav Merrick
2013. ISBN: 978-1-62808-865-6 (Hardcover)
2013. ISBN: 978-1-62808-868-7 (e-book)

Environmental Health Disparities in Children: Asthma, Obesity and Food
Leslie Rubin and Joav Merrick (Editors)
2013. ISBN: 978-1-62948-122-7 (Hardcover)
2013. ISBN: 978-1-62948-135-7 (e-book)

Environmental Health: Home, School and Community
Leslie Rubin and Joav Merrick (Editors)
2013. ISBN: 978-1-62948-155-5 (Hardcover)
2013. ISBN: 978-1-62948-158-6 (e-book)

Guidelines for the Healthy Integration of the Ill Child in the Educational System: Experience from Israel
Yosefa Isenberg
2013. ISBN: 978-1-62808-350-7 (Hardcover)
2013. ISBN: 978-1-62808-353-8 (e-book)

Internet Addiction: A Public Health Concern in Adolescence
Artemis Tsitsika, Mari Janikian, Donald E Greydanus, Hatim A Omar and Joav Merrick (Editors)
2013. ISBN: 978-1-62618-925-6 (Hardcover)
2013. ISBN: 978-1-62618-959-1 (e-book)

Playing with Fire: Children, Adolescents and Firesetting
Hatim A. Omar, Carrie Howell Bowling and Joav Merrick (Editors)
2013. ISBN: 978-1-62948-471-6 (Softcover)
2013. ISBN: 978-1-62948-474-7 (e-book)

Promotion of Holistic Development of Young People in Hong Kong
Daniel TL Shek, Tak Yan Lee and Joav Merrick (Editors)
2013. ISBN: 978-1-62808-019-3 (Hardcover)
2013. ISBN: 978-1-62808-040-7 (e-book)

University and College Students: Health and Development Issues for the Leaders of Tomorrow
Daniel TL Shek, Rachel CF and Joav Merrick (Editors)
2013. ISBN: 978-1-62618-586-9 (Hardcover)
2013. ISBN: 978-1-62618-612-5 (e-book)

Break the Cycle of Environmental Health Disparities: Maternal and Child Health Aspects
Leslie Rubin and Joav Merrick (Editors)
2013. ISBN: 978-1-62948-107-4 (Hardcover)
2013. ISBN: 978-1-62948-133-3 (e-book)

Child and Adolescent Health Yearbook 2012
Joav Merrick (Editor)
2012. ISBN: 978-1-61942-788-4 (Hardcover)
2012. ISBN: 978-1-61942-789-1 (e-book)

Child Health and Human Development Yearbook 2011
Joav Merrick (Editor)
2012. ISBN: 978-1-61942-969-7 (Hardcover)
2012. ISBN: 978-1-61942-970-3 (e-book)

Child and Adolescent Health Yearbook 2011
Joav Merrick (Editor)
2012. ISBN: 978-1-61942-782-2 (Hardcover)
2012. ISBN: 978-1-61942-783-9 (e-book)

Tropical Pediatrics: A Public Health Concern of International Proportions
Richard R Roach, Donald E Greydanus, Dilip R Patel, Douglas N Homnick and Joav Merrick (Editors)
2012. ISBN: 978-1-61942-831-7 (Hardcover)
2012. ISBN: 978-1-61942-840-9 (e-book)

Child Health and Human Development Yearbook 2012
Joav Merrick (Editor)
2012. ISBN: 978-1-61942-978-9 (Hardcover)
2012. ISBN: 978-1-61942-979-6 (e-book)

Developmental Issues in Chinese Adolescents
Daniel TL Shek, Rachel CF Sun and Joav Merrick (Editors)
2012. ISBN: 978-1-62081-262-4 (Hardcover)
2012. ISBN: 978-1-62081-270-9 (e-book)

Positive Youth Development: Theory, Research and Application
Daniel TL Shek, Rachel CF Sun and Joav Merrick (Editors)
2012. ISBN: 978-1-62081-305-8 (Hardcover)
2012. ISBN: 978-1-62081-347-8 (e-book)

Understanding Autism Spectrum Disorder: Current Research Aspects
Ditza A Zachor and Joav Merrick (Editors)
2012. ISBN: 978-1-62081-353-9 (Hardcover)
2012. ISBN: 978-1-62081-390-4 (e-book)

Positive Youth Development: A New School Curriculum to Tackle Adolescent Developmental Issues
Hing Keung Ma, Daniel TL Shek and Joav Merrick (Editors)
2012. ISBN: 978-1-62081-384-3 (Hardcover)
2012. ISBN: 978-1-62081-385-0 (e-book)

Transition from Pediatric to Adult Medical Care
David Wood, John G Reiss, Maria E Ferris, Linda R Edwards and Joav Merrick (Editors)
2012. ISBN: 978-1-62081-409-3 (Hardcover)
2012. ISBN: 978-1-62081-412-3 (e-book)

PEDIATRICS, CHILD AND ADOLESCENT HEALTH

ADOLESCENCE IN CURAÇAO

SORAYA VERSTRAETEN, BAS, MSC
SUPA PENGPID, MPH, DRPH
KARL PELTZER, PHD
AND
JOAV MERRICK, MD, MMEDSCI, DMSC
EDITORS

nova
Medicine & Health
New York

Library of Congress Cataloging-in-Publication Data

Names: Verstraeten, Soraya, editor. | Pengpid, Supa, editor. | Peltzer, Karl, editor. | Merrick, Joav, 1950- editor.
Title: Adolescence in Curaçao / [edited by Soraya Verstraeten, Supa Pengpid, Karl Peltzer, Joav Merrick].
Description: New York : Nova Science Publishers, Inc., [2020] | Series: Pediatrics, child and adolescent health | Includes bibliographical references and index. |
Identifiers: LCCN 2020005571 (print) | LCCN 2020005572 (ebook) | ISBN 9781536175226 (paperback) | ISBN 9781536175233 (adobe pdf)
Subjects: LCSH: Teenagers--Health and hygiene--Curaçao.
Classification: LCC RA564.5 .A325 2020 (print) | LCC RA564.5 (ebook) | DDC 613/.04330972986--dc23
LC record available at https://lccn.loc.gov/2020005571
LC ebook record available at https://lccn.loc.gov/2020005572

Published by Nova Science Publishers, Inc. † New York

CONTENTS

INTRODUCTION

In: Adolescence in Curaçao
Editors: Soraya Verstraeten et al.
ISBN: 978-1-53617-522-6

Chapter 1

GLOBAL SCHOOL-BASED STUDENT HEALTH SURVEY IN CURAÇAO

Soraya Verstraeten[1], MSc,
Supa Pengpid[2,3,*], DrPH, Karl Peltzer[3], PhD
and Joav Merrick[4-7], MD, MMedSci, DMSc

[1]Institute for Public Health (Volksgezondheid Instituut Curaçao),
Ministry of Public Health, Environment and Nature,
Willemstad, Curaçao
[2]ASEAN Institute for Health Development, Mahidol University,
Salaya, Phutthamonthon, Nakhon Pathom, Thailand
[3]Department of Research Administration and Development,
University of Limpopo, Turfloop, South Africa
[4]National Institute of Child Health and Human Development,
Jerusalem, Israel
[5]Department of Pediatrics, Mt. Scopus Campus,
Hadassah Hebrew University Medical Center,
Jerusalem, Israel

* ***Correspondence***: supaprom@yahoo.com.

[6]Kentucky Children's Hospital, University of Kentucky,
Lexington, Kentucky, United States of America
[7]Center for Healthy Development, School of Public Health,
Georgia State University, Atlanta, United States of America

ABSTRACT

In this book we present research from the Curaçao "Global School-based Student Health Survey" (GSHS). The World Health Organization (WHO) and United States "Centers for Disease Control and Prevention (CDC)" in their collaboration around this survey help countries to assess ten behavioural risk and protective factors, including alcohol use, dietary behaviours, drug use, hygiene, mental health, physical activity, protective factors, sexual behaviours, tobacco use, violence and unintentional injury among adolescents. In the survey a self-administered questionnaire is used to obtain data on young people's health behaviour and protective factors related to the leading causes of morbidity and mortality among children and adults worldwide. We hope that the results from this survey in Curaçao will inform stakeholders of the importance of a healthy school environment, for setting priorities, establishing programmes, and advocating for school and youth health programmes and related policies.

INTRODUCTION

The "Global School-based Student Health Survey (GSHS)" is a World Health Organization (WHO) and United States "Centers for Disease Control and Prevention (CDC)" collaborative effort in helping countries to assess ten behavioural risk and protective factors, including "alcohol use, dietary behaviours, drug use, hygiene, mental health, physical activity, protective factors, sexual behaviours, tobacco use, violence and unintentional injury" among adolescents [1]. "The GSHS is a relatively low-cost school-based survey which uses a self-administered questionnaire to obtain data on young people's health behaviour and protective factors related to the leading causes of morbidity and mortality among children and adults worldwide" [1].

Apart from countries in Africa, Eastern Europe, Eastern Mediterranean, Southeast Asia, Western Pacific that participated in the GSHS, various countries in the Americas and the Caribbean, including countries, such as Bahamas, Barbados, British Virgin Islands, Cayman Islands, Dominica, Dominican Republic and Grenada have also embarked on their national GSHS.

Curaçao has now also embarked on the GSHS joining a large number of countries. Curaçao is a high-income Caribbean island country with about 159,000 inhabitants, mainly of African descent (75.4%) [2].

In this book we present research from the Curaçao GSHS sponsored by the Ministry of Health, Nature and Environment in Curaçao. The results of the various papers will inform stakeholders of the importance of a healthy school environment, for setting priorities, establishing programmes, and advocating for school and youth health programmes and related policies [3].

ACKNOWLEDGMENTS

This book is an adapted version of papers published in the special issue of the International Public Health Journal 2020; 12(3) on "Global School-Based Student Health Survey in Curaçao" edited by Soraya Verstraeten, Supa Pengpid, Karl Peltzer and Joav Merrick.

REFERENCES

[1] World Health Organization (WHO) Global school-based student health survey (GSHS). URL: https://www.who.int/ncds/surveillance/ gshs/en/.

[2] Pan American Health Organization. Country report: Curaçao, 2017. *URL*: https://www.paho.org/salud-en-las-americas-2017/ ?page_id=141.

[3] Verstraeten, S. The Curaçao Global School-based Student Health Survey (GSHS). Willemstad: Volksgezondheid Instituut Curaçao, 2015.

SECTION ONE: GLOBAL SCHOOL-BASED STUDENT HEALTH SURVEY

In: Adolescence in Curaçao
Editors: Soraya Verstraeten et al.
ISBN: 978-1-53617-522-6

Chapter 2

PREVALENCE AND CORRELATES OF SEXUAL RISK BEHAVIOUR AMONG A NATIONAL SAMPLE OF SCHOOL-GOING ADOLESCENTS IN CURAÇAO

Soraya Verstraeten[1], MSc, Supa Pengpid[2,3,*], DrPH and Karl Peltzer[3], PhD

[1]Institute for Public Health (Volksgezondheid Instituut Curaçao), Ministry of Public Health, Environment and Nature, Willemstad, Curaçao

[2]ASEAN Institute for Health Development, Mahidol University, Salaya, Phutthamonthon, Nakhon Pathom, Thailand

[3]Department of Research Administration and Development, University of Limpopo, Turfloop, South Africa

[*] ***Correspondence***: Professor Supa Pengpid, ASEAN Institute for Health Development, Mahidol University, 25/25 Phutthamonthon Road 4, Salaya, Phutthamonton, Nakhon Pathom 73170, Thailand. Email: supaprom@yahoo.com.

ABSTRACT

In this chapter we aim to assess the prevalence and correlates of sexual risk behaviour among school-going adolescents in Curaçao. In the cross-sectional Curaçao "Global School-Based Student Health Survey (GSHS)" in 2015, 2,765 adolescents (median age 15 years) responded to questions on sociodemographic factors, substance use, interpersonal violence, psychological distress, protective factors and sexual risk behaviour. Of students who ever had sex (35.5%), 24.0% had early sexual debut, 51.3% had multiple sexual partners, 39.3% had not used a condom at last sex, and on average engaged in 2.2 sexual risk behaviours. In multivariable logistic regression analysis, male sex for ever sex and multiple sexual partners, female sex for non-condom use at last sex, older age, heavy alcohol use, tobacco use, in a physical fight, carried a weapon, physical partner violence, and school truancy were associated with ≥ two and/or multiple sexual risk behaviours. Our results suggest that Curaçaoan adolescent's need increased access to comprehensive sexual and reproductive education and health service that integrate substance use, interpersonal violence prevention, mental health and parental education. Moreover, programmes improving school attendance and preventing school truancy can help in reducing sexual risk behaviours.

INTRODUCTION

The onset of sexual activity often falls within the period of adolescence and is frequently associated with sexual risk behaviour, including the lack of condom and contraceptive use (1). In several Caribbean countries, a high prevalence of ever sex, non-condom use, and non-contraceptive use have been found in adolescent populations. In Haiti, 60% of 13- to 18-year old adolescents had experienced sexual intercourse, and boys were far more likely to participate in early sexual debut (<14 years old), multiple sex partners, and non-condom use, than girls (2). In Jamaica, 79% of 15- to 24-year olds reported ever sex (mean age 14.7 years), and among those sexually active, a large proportion engaged in inconsistent condom use (59%), multiple sex partners (45%) and transactional sex (43%) (3). In Anguilla, sexual activity was associated with male gender, recent substance use, recent depression and a history of physical and sexual abuse (4).

Sexual violence is a pervasive concern in the region: in nine Caribbean countries, almost half (48%) of the adolescent girls that ever had sex reported that their first intercourse was (somewhat) forced (5). Another cross-country study covering data from 6 Caribbean countries found that early onset of sexual behaviour (<15 years old) is relatively high among 13-to 16-year old Caribbean adolescents (27%), and is associated with male gender, tobacco and alcohol use, having been in a physical fight, sedentary behaviour, truancy and lack of parental or guardian attachment (6). High-risk sexual risk behaviours such as early sexual debut, inconsistent condom use, and having multiple sexual partners were previously identified as common risk factors for sexual transmitted diseases among Jamaican adolescents (7, 8). Relatedly, the "Caribbean is the second most-affected region in the world in terms of HIV prevalence rates," with 1% of the adult population infected (9).

There is lack of information on the prevalence and correlates of sexual risk behaviour among adolescents in Curaçao, a high-income Dutch Caribbean island. The scarce data available on sexually transmitted diseases and other negative consequences of sexual behaviour indicate that sexual risk behaviour are a matter of concern in Curaçao as well. In 2015, 13 new HIV-infections were registered among 15-to-24 year olds, and the positivity rate for Chlamydia trachomatis among this age group was 25% (10). Adolescent pregnancy rates decreased but are still high compared other Caribbean countries and the Netherlands (11, 12), often resulting in unwanted pregnancies, abortion, school dropout and low school attainment (13, 14). To better tailor policy interventions aimed at improving the sexual health behaviours that underly the high rates of sexually transmitted diseases, pregnancies and abortions among adolescents in Curaçao, this study aims to provide a better insight in the prevalence and correlates of sexual risk behaviour among Curaçaoan adolescents.

OUR STUDY

Cross-sectional data from the 2015 Curaçao GSHS were analyzed (15). The study used a two-stage cluster sample design to produce data representative of all students enrolled in public secondary education, comparable to US Grades 1-6, in Curaçao. "At the first stage, 28 schools were selected with probability proportional to enrolment size, and at the second stage, 161 classes were randomly selected" (16). All students in selected classes were eligible to participate after ethical approval *in accordance with the "WMA Declaration of Helsinki – Ethical Principles for Medical Research Involving Human Subjects"* and other permissions were granted and informed consent was obtained from parents and children; the overall response rate was 83% (16).

Measures

The dataset from the self-administered GSHS questionnaire was used in this study (15). The four outcome variables included: 1) sexual initiation during adolescence, 2) early age of sexual debut, 3) two or more sexual partners in a lifetime, and 4) no condom use at last sex. A description of the independent variables and their coding is depicted in Appendix 1. The four questions on parental or guardian support were summed up and categorized into 0-1 low, 2 medium and 3-4 high support. Psychological distress was defined as zero, single as one and multiple as 2-5 psychological distress items of 1) no close friends, 2) loneliness, 3) anxiety, 4) suicidal ideation and 5) suicide attempt.

Data analysis

Data analysis was conducted with STATA software version 15.0 (Stata Corporation, College Station, TX, USA), taking into account the complex study design. Chi-square tests were used to test differences in proportions.

Multivariable logistic and linear regression was used to assess the associations between independent variables (sociodemographic factors, substance use, interpersonal violence, psychological distress, and protective factors) and four individual sexual risk behaviours (ever had sex, early sexual debut, multiple sexual partners, and non-condom use at last sex) and a composite measure of the four sexual risk behaviours. Missing data were excluded from the analysis. P values <0.05 were considered significant.

FINDINGS

The sample consisted of 2765 school-going adolescents (median age 15 years), 51.1% female and 48.9% male, 3.8% had mostly or always experienced hunger in the past month, 81.7% had parents or guardians that provided them mostly or always with necessities, and 69.0% perceived themselves to be a religious or spiritual person. More than one-third of the students (35.5%) ever had sex, and among sexually active students, 24.0% had an early sexual debut (<15 years), 51.3% had two or more (multiple) sexual partners, 39.3% had not used a condom at last sex. On average, sexually active students engaged in 2.2 (SD=0.9) sexual risk behaviours. Students' reports of all sexual risk behaviours, except early sexual debut, increased with age. Boys engaged more often than girls in ever had sex (P<0.001), early sexual debut (P<0.001), and multiple sexual partners (P<0.001), while girls had a high proportion of non-condom use at last sex (P<0.001). Sex differences for the sexual risk composite score were non-significant (P=0.187) (see Table 1).

Table 1. Sample characteristics and sexual risk behaviour

Variable	Total	Ever sex	Early sexual debut[1]	Multiple sex partners[1]	No condom last sex[1]	Sexual risk composite score[1]
	N (%)	%	%	%	%	M (SD)
All	2765	35.5	24.0	51.3	39.3	2.2 (0.9)
Sociodemographics						
Age in years						
≤11-14	1054 (32.8)	15.2	44.4	22.4	24.0	1.9 (1.0)
15-16	824 (32.7)	33.4	27.7	47.8	38.5	2.2 (1.0)
17-18 or more	877 (34.5)	64.3	18.0	59.1	42.8	2.2 (0.9)
Sex						
Female	1508 (51.1)	35.7	16.9	47.2	49.8	2.1 (0.9)
Male	1230 (48.9)	41.5	30.6	55.1	29.3	2.1 (1.0)
Parents provide necessities	2082 (81.7)	36.6	22.0	50.7	39.3	2.1 (0.9)
Experience hunger	102 (3.8)	46.3	35.1	56.5	34.4	2.3 (1.0)
Religious or spiritual person	1717 (69.0)	37.7	22.5	52.4	40.3	2.2 (0.9)
Substance use						
Current tobacco use	345 (13.2)	65.3	28.2	63.4	43.1	2.3 (0.9)
Heavy alcohol use	477 (19.0)	65.0	28.2	63.5	46.3	2.4 (0.9)
Current cannabis use	136 (5.7)	62.8	31.3	65.3	50.6	2.5 (1.0)
Ever amphetamine, cocaine, etc. use	45 (1.7)	71.6	45.0	67.5	57.1	2.7 (0.9)
Interpersonal violence						
In physical fight	492 (17.9)	48.6	20.4	51.5	37.9	2.3 (1.0)
Carried a weapon	363 (13.9)	59.2	31.7	58.2	39.0	2.3 (0.9)
Belongs to violent group	165 (6.1)	50.1	36.0	64.7	45.7	2.5 (0.8)
Partner violence	282 (10.2)	51.0	31.7	61.3	48.2	2.4 (1.0)

Variable	Total	Ever sex	Early sexual debut[1]	Multiple sex partners[1]	No condom last sex[1]	Sexual risk composite score[1]
	N (%)	%	%	%	%	M (SD)
Psychological distress						
0	1719 (65.1)	35.3	21.7	53.2	36.4	2.1 (0.9)
1	531 (20.5)	37.3	24.3	47.9	38.6	2.1 (0.9)
2-5	379 (14.4)	54.1	28.4	49.6	49.9	2.3 (0.9)
Protective factors						
Has heard about HIV or AIDS	1948 (76.9)	39.8	23.6	54.4	39.5	2.2 (0.9)
Was taught about avoiding HIV/AIDS	1301 (51.0)	40.6	23.6	51.3	39.5	2.1 (0.9)
Ever talked about HIV/AIDS with parents	1233 (48.5)	42.0	22.2	50.4	38.1	2.1 (0.9)
School attendance	1976 (73.4)	31.9	21.2	47.6	35.8	2.0 (0.9)
Peer support	1241 (47.6)	38.7	21.4	52.0	40.1	2.1 (1.0)
Lives with both parents	1325 (48.9)	32.5	20.1	47.2	35.0	2.0 (0.9)
Parental support						
Low	665 (27.2)	51.7	27.6	54.1	42.2	2.2 (1.0)
Medium	659 (26.7)	37.9	23.7	54.0	38.9	2.2 (1.0)
High	1167 (46.1)	31.1	20.7	48.7	37.2	2.1 (0.9)

[1]Of sexually active students.

Associations between sexual risk behaviour and independent variables

Results from the multivariable regression analysis verify the associations between age, sex and sexual risks behaviours from the descriptive statistics. The indicators of socioeconomic status (parental provision of necessities and the experience of hunger) and the perception of being a religious or spiritual person were not significantly associated with any of the four sexual risk behaviours and the sexual risk composite score.

Regarding substance use, heavy alcohol use (≥2 drinks/day) was associated with all four sexual risk behaviors and the sexual risk composite score, and current tobacco use was associated with ever sex, multiple sexual partners and the sexual risk composite score. Considering interpersonal violence, being in a physical fight, carrying a weapon and experiencing partner violence were associated with two or three of the individual sexual risk behaviours and all three forms of violence were associated with the sexual risk composite score. In contrast, belonging to a violent group (or gang) was not significantly associated with sexual risk behaviours. Multiple psychological distress was associated with ever sex and non-condom use at last sex.

The strongest protective factors were school attendance and living with both parents, which were both negatively associated with all four sexual risk behaviours and the sexual risk composite score. Higher parental support was protective from ever having sex and the sexual risk composite score. Having heard of HIV/AIDS was associated with early sexual debut, having multiple sexual partners and the sexual risk composite score. Having ever talked about HIV/AIDS with their parents or guardians was protective from having multiple sexual partners, and having been taught about how to avoid HIV/AIDS in the past year was not associated with any sexual risk behaviours (see Table 2).

Table 2. Estimated association between sociodemographics, substance use, interpersonal violence, psychological distress and protective factors with sexual risk behaviors

Variable	Ever sex	Early sexual debut	Multiple sexual partners	No condom at last sex	Sexual risk composite
	Unadjusted OR (95% CI)	Unadjusted OR (95% CI)	Unadjusted OR (95% CI)	Unadjusted OR (95% CI)	Exp (Coef.) (95% CI)
Sociodemographics					
Age in years					
≤11-14	1 (Reference)	1 (Reference)	1 (Reference)	1 (Reference)	Reference
15-16	3.05 (2.10, 4.42)***	1.37 (0.79, 2.36)	6.89 (3.61, 13.16)***	4.90 (2.67, 9.00)***	1.43 (1.25, 1.64)***
17-18 or more	10.92 (7.49, 15.95)***	1.58 (0.90, 2.78)	21.75 (13.51, 35.02)***	11.88 (6.96, 20.31)***	2.55 (2.24, 2.91)***
Sex					
Female	1 (Reference)	1 (Reference)	1 (Reference)	1 (Reference)	Reference
Male	1.40 (1.28, 2.85)**	2.60 (1.77, 3.81)***	1.52 (1.02, 2.28)*	0.55 (0.41, 0.73)***	1.10 (1.00, 1.21)
Parents provide necessities	0.74 (0.54, 1.01)	0.70 (0.43, 1.15)	0.83 (0.63, 1.31)	0.94 (0.70, 1.43)	0.90 (0.74, 1.09)
Experience hunger	0.88 (0.43, 1.84)	1.48 (0.81, 2.70)	0.81 (0.31, 2.14)	0.82 (0.37, 1.84)	0.97 (0.73, 1.29)
Religious or spiritual person	1.01 (0.77, 1.32)	0.89 (0.59, 1.35)	1.42 (0.96, 2.10)	1.00 (0.70, 1.49)	1.03 (0.91, 1.18)
Substance use					
Current tobacco use	1.91 (1.28, 2.85)**	1.41 (0.82, 2.41)	1.83 (1.19, 2.84)**	1.28 (0.77, 2.11)	1.33 (1.08, 1.64)**
Heavy alcohol use	1.76 (1.32, 2.34)***	1.71 (1.11, 2.64)*	1.51 (1.02, 2.22)*	1.70 (1.28, 2.26)***	1.41 (1.23, 1.62)***
Current cannabis use	0.73 (0.38, 1.40)	0.71 (0.30, 1.70)	1.64 (0.73, 3.69)	0.84 (0.41, 1.73)	0.94 (0.68, 1.31)
Ever amphetamine, cocaine, etc. use	1.02 (0.33, 3.17)	0.93 (0.28, 3.08)	1.00 (0.21, 4.81)	1.04 (0.42, 2.57)	1.08 (0.66, 1.77)
Interpersonal violence					
In physical fight	1.80 (1.29, 2.53)***	2.26 (1.55, 3.30)***	1.83 (1.32, 2.52)***	1.58 (0.98, 2.54)	1.32 (1.15, 1.51)***
Carried a weapon	1.98 (1.40, 2.80)***	1.40 (0.94, 2.09)	1.63 (1.13, 2.36)**	1.28 (0.74, 2.22)	1.33 (1.13, 1.57)***

Table 2. (Continued)

Variable	Ever sex	Early sexual debut	Multiple sexual partners	No condom at last sex	Sexual risk composite
	Unadjusted OR (95% CI)	Unadjusted OR (95% CI)	Unadjusted OR (95% CI)	Unadjusted OR (95% CI)	Exp (Coef.) (95% CI)
Belongs to violent group	1.11 (0.60, 2.02)	1.41 (0.69, 2.87)	1.77 (0.82, 3.84)	1.58 (0.78, 3.21)	1.20 (0.92, 1.56)
Partner violence	1.33 (0.94, 1.89)	2.09 (1.17, 3.73)*	1.60 (1.15, 2.22)**	1.78 (1.20, 2.65)**	1.38 (1.16, 1.67)***
Psychological distress					
0	1 (Reference)	1 (Reference)	1 (Reference)	1 (Reference)	Reference
1	0.73 (0.53, 1.01)	0.92 (0.53, 1.59)	0.62 (0.42, 0.89)*	0.87 (0.57, 1.32)	0.86 (0.76, 0.97)*
2-5	1.48 (1.00, 2.19)*	1.09 (0.69, 1.71)	0.95 (0.56, 1.61)	1.66 (1.09, 2.54)*	1.11 (0.92, 1.33)
Protective factors					
Has heard about HIV or AIDS	1.05 (0.80, 1.37)	1.74 (1.08, 2.83)*	1.96 (1.24, 3.09)**	1.22 (0.77, 1.93)	1.12 (1.01, 1.24)*
Was taught about avoiding HIV/AIDS	1.16 (0.91, 1.49)	1.01 (0.68, 1.50)	1.19 (0.87, 1.63)	1.14 (0.81, 1.60)	1.07 (0.95, 1.19)
Ever talked about HIV/AIDS with parents	1.27 (0.98, 1.64)	1.08 (0.78, 1.51)	0.71 (0.52, 0.98)*	0.90 (0.67, 1.22)	1.02 (0.93, 1.13)
School attendance	0.54 (0.43, 0.69)***	0.52 (0.37, 0.74)***	0.57 (0.42, 0.79)***	0.68 (0.52, 0.92)*	0.74 (0.64, 0.84)***
Peer support	1.12 (0.89. 1.41)	0.98 (0.70, 1.38)	1.01 (0.76, 1.35)	1.18 (0.83, 1.66)	1.05 (0.96, 1.16)
Lives with both parents	0.67 (0.53, 0.84)***	0.58 (0.42, 0.80)***	0.68 (0.48, 0.95)*	0.67 (0.47, 0.95)*	0.81 (0.74, 0.90)****
Parental support					
Low	1 (Reference)	1 (Reference)	1 (Reference)	1 (Reference)	Reference
Medium	0.67 (0.50, 0.90)**	0.75 (0.43, 1.33)	0.80 (0.53, 1.22)	0.82 (0.57, 1.19)	0.85 (0.73, 0.99)*
High	0.71 (0.54, 0.96)*	0.77 (0.46, 1.28)	0.78 (0.56, 1.09)	0.76 (0.57, 1.02)	0.86 (0.75, 0.98)*

Unadjusted OR=Unadjusted Odds Ratio; ***P<0.001; **P<0.01; *P<0.05.

DISCUSSION

The study found a prevalence of ever had sex of 35.5% among a representative sample of school-going adolescents in Curaçao. Among sexually active students, this study found a high prevalence of individual sexual risk behaviours (early sexual debut 24.0%, multiple sexual partners 51.3%, and non-condom use at last sex 39.3%). On average, sexually active students engaged in 2.2 (SD=0.9) sexual risk behaviours. In comparison to results among adolescents in 15 other Caribbean countries, students in Curaçao were less likely to report they ever had sex and early debut, but condom use during last sex was average (16). Socio-cultural factors, such as a cultural taboo on talking about sex, negative attitudes towards condom use and limited knowledge about contraception and sexual health, have been previously been implicated as contributing factors to inconsistent condom use in Curaçao (14, 17, 18).

Male sex was associated with ever had sex, early sexual debut and multiple sex partners, while female sex was associated with non-condom use during last sex. This shows that female students in Curaçao are more vulnerable to HIV infection, possibly by having relationships with older men who are more likely to have contracted the virus (19). These findings suggest that adolescent's need access to comprehensive sexual and reproductive education and health services.

In agreement with a number of previous studies in non-Caribbean countries, substance use (tobacco, alcohol) was highly associated with sexual risk behaviours and multiple sexual risk behaviours (20-24). In addition, psychological distress, in particular multiple psychological distress was associated with some sexual risk behaviours, which was also found in previous studies (20, 22, 25-27). These findings seem to suggest a clustering of substance use, interpersonal violence and psychological distress with sexual risk behaviour, calling for sexual health programmes that integrate substance use, violence prevention and mental health (20-22).

School attendance was protective from all sexual risk behaviours and multiple sexual risk behaviours, which confirms findings from previous investigations (20, 21, 26). This result could mean that programmes improving school attendance and preventing school truancy can help in reducing sexual risk behaviours. Previous studies found that parental support was protective from sexual risk behaviours (2, 21, 25, 26), while in this study high parental or guardian support was protective from ever had sex but not with any of the other sexual risk behaviours. As parents and guardians act as "primary socializing agents who strongly influence their adolescents' behaviours and expectancies regarding timing and involvement in sexual behaviors and relationships" (28), this may imply that family-focused education campaigns targeting sexual risk behaviour is wanted.

Study limitations

The GSHS is limited to participants attending high schools in the public education system, which does not include out-off school adolescents and students in the private education system. The questionnaire was administered by self-report, and therefore some of the responses may have been biased; sexual behaviour, especially among females, may have been underreported. The survey data were cross-sectional; no causal conclusions can be drawn from our results.

CONCLUSION

More than one third of school-going adolescents ever had sex, and among sexually active a high prevalence of sexual risk behaviours (early sexual debut, multiple sexual partners, and non-condom use during last sex) was found. School truancy, living with only one or no parent, substance use (heavy drinking and tobacco), interpersonal violence (in physical fight, carrying a weapon and physical partner violence) and psychological distress were associated with individual and multiple sexual risk behaviours. Our results suggest that adolescent's need increased access to comprehensive sexual and reproductive education and health services in Curaçao that integrate substance use, interpersonal violence prevention, mental health and parental education. Moreover, programs improving school attendance and preventing school truancy can help in reducing sexual risk behaviors.

APPENDIX 1. DESCRIPTION OF INDEPENDENT VARIABLES USED IN THIS STUDY

Variables	Question	Response options (Coding scheme)
	Sociodemographic factors	
Age	"How old are you?"	"11 years old or younger to 18 years old or older"
Sex	"What is your sex?"	"Male, Female"
Provision of necessities	"During the past 30 days, how often did your parents or guardians provide for your necessities?"	"1= never to 5= always (coded 1–3=0 and 4–5=1)"
Hunger	"During the past 30 days, how often did you go hungry because there was not enough food in your home?"	"1= never to 5= always (coded 1–3=0 and 4–5=1)"
Religious or spiritual person	"Do you think of yourself as a religious or spiritual person?"	"Yes, No"
	Substance use	
Current tobacco use	"During the past 30 days, on how many days did you smoke cigarettes/use any tobacco products other than cigarettes, such as cigars, cigarillos, or electronic cigarettes?"	"1=0 days to 7=All 30 days (coded 1=0 and 2-7=1)"
Heavy alcohol use (2 or more/day)	"During the past 30 days, on the days you drink alcohol, how many drinks did you usually drink per day?"	"1 = Not drink in the past 30 days to 7 = 5 or more drinks (coded 1–3 = 0 and 4–7 = 1)"
Current cannabis use	"During the past 30 days, how many times have you used marijuana (also called weed, pot, cannabis, ganja, or grass)?"	"1=0 days to 7=All 30 days (coded 1=0 and 2-7=1)"
Lifetime methamphetamine, etc. use	"During your life, how many times have you used methamphetamine, cocaine, or XTC (also called speed, base, rock, crack, and uppers)?"	"1=0 times to 5=20 or more times (coded 1=0 and 2-5=1)"

Appendix 1. (Continued)

Variables	Question	Response options (Coding scheme)
	Interpersonal violence	
In a physical fight	"During the past 12 months, how many times were you in a physical fight?"	"1=0 times to 8=12 or more times (coded 1=0 and 2–8=1)"
Carried a weapon	"During the past 30 days, on how many days did you carry a weapon, such as a gun, knife, club, or brass knuckles?"	"1=0 days to 5=6 or more days) (coded 1=0 and 2-6=1)"
Belong to violent group	"Do you belong to any violent group?"	"Yes, No"
Partner violence	"During the past 12 months, did your boyfriend or girlfriend ever hit, slap, or physically hurt you on purpose?"	"Yes, No"
	Psychological distress	
No close friends	"How many close friends do you have?"	"1 = 0 to 4 = 3 or more (coded 1+=0, 0=1)"
Anxiety	"During the past 12 months, how often have you been so worried about something that you could not sleep at night?"	"1=never to 5=always (coded 1–3=0 and 4–5=1)"
Loneliness	"During the past 12 months, how often have you felt lonely?"	"1=never to 5=always (coded 1–3=0 and 4–5=1)"
Suicide ideation	"During the past 12 months, did you ever seriously consider attempting suicide?"	"Yes, No"
Suicide attempt	"During the past 12 months, how many times did you actually attempt suicide?"	"1=0 times to 5=6 or more times (coded 1=0 and 2–5=1)"
	Protective factors	
Heard about HIV/AIDS	"Have you ever heard of HIV infection or the disease called AIDS?"	"Yes, No"
Was taught about avoiding HIV/AIDS	"During this school year, were you taught in any of your classes how to avoid HIV infection or AIDS?"	"Yes, No"
Ever talked about HIV/AIDS with parents	"Have you ever talked about HIV infection or AIDS with your parents or guardians?"	"Yes, No"
School attendance	"During the past 30 days, on how many days did you miss classes or school without permission?"	"1=0 days to 5= 10 or more days (coded 1=0 and 2–5=1)"

Variables	Question	Response options (Coding scheme)
	Protective factors	
Peer support	"During the past 30 days, how often were most of the students in your school kind and helpful?"	"1=never to 5=always (coded 1–3=0 and 4–5=1)"
Lives with both parents	"Which adult family members do you live with?"	"1=both my mother and father to 5=I do not live with any adult family members (coded 2-5=0 and 1=1)"
Parental supervision	"During the past 30 days, how often did your parents or guardians check to see if your homework was done?"	"1=never to 5=always (coded 1–3=0 and 4–5=1)"
Parental connectedness	"During the past 30 days, how often did your parents or guardians understand your problems and worries?"	"1=never to 5=always (coded 1–3=0 and 4–5=1)"
Parental bonding	"During the past 30 days, how often did your parents or guardians really know what you were doing with your free time?	"1=never to 5=always (coded 1–3=0 and 4–5=1)"
Parental respect for privacy	"During the past 30 days, how often did your parents or guardians go through your things without your approval?"	"1=never to 5=always (coded 1–3=0 and 4–5=1)"

REFERENCES

[1] Bearinger LH, Sieving RE, Ferguson J, Sharma V. Global perspectives on the sexual and reproductive health of adolescents: patterns, prevention, and potential. Lancet 2007;369:1220-31.

[2] Carver JW, Dévieux JG, Gaston SC, Altice FL, Niccolai LM. Sexual risk behaviors among adolescents in Port-au-Prince, Haiti. AIDS Behav 2014;18(8):1595–603.

[3] Jarrett SB, Udell W, Sutherland S, McFarland W, Scott M, Skyers N. Age at sexual initiation and sexual and health risk behaviors among Jamaican adolescents and young adults. AIDS Behav 2018;22(Suppl 1):57–64.

[4] Kurtz SP, Douglas KG, Lugo Y. Sexual risks and concerns about AIDS among adolescents in Anguilla. AIDS Care 2005;17(Suppl 1):S36-44.

[5] Halcón L, Blum RW, Beuhring T, Pate E, Campbell-Forrester S, Venema A. Adolescent health in the Caribbean: a regional portrait. Am J Public Health 2003;93(11):1851–7.

[6] Peltzer K, Pengpid S. Early Sexual debut and associated factors among in-school adolescents in six Caribbean countries. West Indian Med J 2015;64(4):351–6.
[7] Smikle MF, Dowe G, Hylton-Kong T, Williams E, Baum M. Risky behaviour in Jamaican adolescent patients attending a sexually transmitted disease clinic. West Indian Med J 2000;49(4):327–30.
[8] Normann LR. Sexually transmitted disease symptoms: A comparative analysis of male and female youth in Jamaica. West Indian Med J 2001;50(3):203–8.
[9] UNAIDS. Miles to go. The response to HIV in the Caribbean. Geneva, Switzerland: UNAIDS, 2018.
[10] Volksgezondheid Instituut Curaçao. De Gezondheidsdatabank Curaçao, 2016. URL: www.vic.cw.
[11] van Enk WJ, Gorissen WH, van Enk A. Teenage pregnancy and ethnicity in The Netherlands: frequency and obstetric outcome. Eur J Contracept Reprod Health Care 2000;5(1):77–84.
[12] Volksgezondheid Instituut Curaçao. Factsheet tienermoeders, 2015. URL: www.vic.cw.
[13] Boersma A, Alberts J, Bruijn J De, Meyboom BJ, Kleiverda G. Termination of pregnancy in Curaçao: need for improvement of sexual and reproductive healthcare. Glob J Health Sci 2012;4(3):30–8.
[14] Hellings E. Jong (&) Moeder. Willemstad, Curaçao; 2010. URL: http://www.faj.cw/index.php?topic=onderzoeksrapporten.
[15] World Health Organization (WHO). Global School-based Student Health Survey (GSHS). URL: http://www.who.int/chp/gshs/en/.
[16] Verstraeten S. The Curaçao Global School-based Student Health Survey (GSHS). Willemstad: Volksgezondheid Instituut Curaçao, 2015.
[17] Stutterheim SE, Bertens MGBC, Mevissen FEF, Schaalma HP. Factors contributing to inconsistent condom use among heterosexual men in Curaçao. Cult Health Sex 2013;15(4):420–33.
[18] van den Brink MJ, Boersma AA, Meyboom-de Jong B, de Bruijn JGM. Attitude toward contraception and abortion among Curaçao women. Ineffective contraception due to limited sexual education? BMC Fam Pract 2011;12(1):55.
[19] UNICEF. The situation of children and adolescents in Curaçao: key findings and recommendations, 2013. URL: https://www.unicef.nl/media/1371768/Curaçao_executive_summary__28english_29.pdf.
[20] Peltzer K, Pengpid S. Risk and protective factors affecting sexual risk behavior among school-aged adolescents in Fiji, Kiribati, Samoa, and Vanuatu. Asia Pacific J Public Health 2016;28(5):404–15.
[21] Mmari K, Blum RW. Risk and protective factors that affect adolescent reproductive health in developing countries: A structured literature review. Glob Public Health 2009;4:350–66.

[22] Page RM, Hall CP. Psychosocial distress and alcohol use as factors in adolescent sexual behavior among sub-saharan african adolescents. J Sch Health 2009;79:369–79.

[23] Liu A, Kilmarx P, Jenkins RA, Manopaiboon C, Mock PA, Jeeyapunt S, et al. Sexual initiation, substance use, and sexual behavior and knowledge among vocational students in Northern Thailand. Int Fam Plan Perspect 2006;32:126–35.

[24] Siziya S, Muula AS, Kazembe LN, Rudatsikira E. Harmful lifestyles' clustering among sexually active in-school adolescents in Zambia. BMC Pediatr 2008;8:1–7.

[25] Peltzer K, Pengpid S. Prevalence and social correlates of sexual intercourse among school-going adolescents in Thailand. ScientificWorldJournal 2011;11:1812–20.

[26] Ahmad NA, Awaluddin SM, Ismail H, Samad R, NikAbdRashid NR. Sexual activity among Malaysian school-going adolescents: what are the risk and protective factors? Asia Pac J Public Health 2014;26(5 Suppl):44S-52S.

[27] Peltzer K. Early sexual debut and associated factors among in-school adolescents in eight African countries. Acta Paediatr 2010;99:1242–7.

[28] Coley RL, Votruba-Drzal E, Schindler HS. Fathers' and mothers' parenting predicting and responding to adolescent sexual risk behaviors. Child Dev 2009;80(3):808–27.

In: Adolescence in Curaçao
Editors: Soraya Verstraeten et al.
ISBN: 978-1-53617-522-6

Chapter 3

RISK AND PROTECTIVE FACTORS OF ADOLESCENT PREGNANCY IN CURAÇAO

Soraya Verstraeten*[1], *MSc*, *Supa Pengpid*[2,3,*], *DrPH* and *Karl Peltzer*[3], *PhD

[1]Institute for Public Health (Volksgezondheid Instituut Curaçao), Ministry of Public Health, Environment and Nature, Willemstad, Curaçao
[2]ASEAN Institute for Health Development, Mahidol University, Salaya, Phutthamonthon, Nakhon Pathom, Thailand
[3]Department of Research Administration and Development, University of Limpopo, Turfloop, South Africa

ABSTRACT

In this chapter we wanted to assess risk and protective factors among school-going adolescent girls in Curaçao. In the cross-sectional Curaçao "Global School-Based Student Health Survey (GSHS)" in 2015, 1,508 female students (median age 16 years) responded to questions on pregnancy, sociodemographic factors, risk and protective factors of adolescent

---

[*] ***Correspondence***: Professor Supa Pengpid, ASEAN Institute for Health Development, Mahidol University, 25/25 Phutthamonthon Road 4, Salaya, Phutthamonton, Nakhon Pathom 73170, Thailand. Email: supaprom@yahoo.com.

pregnancy. In all, 5.8% of female students reported to have been pregnant. In adjusted logistic regression analysis, having had multiple sexual partners was positively and parental provision of necessities was negatively associated with adolesecent pregnancy. In addition, in unadjusted analysis, early sexual debut, transactional sex, history of forced sexual intercourse, physical intimate partner violence victimization, substance use, psychological distress were associated with adolescent pregnancy, and school attendance and high parental support were protective from adolescent pregnancy. One in seventen girls reported adolescent pregnancy and the knowledge of the identified risk factors can assist in tailoring prevention strategies. Knowledge of the identified risk factors, such as low parental provision of necessities and having multiple sexual partners, can assist in tailoring pregnancy prevention programmes.

INTRODUCTION

Adolescent girls are vulnerable because they face the risks of unplanned pregnancy and childbirth, often in a context with limited access to contraception and services for pregnancy support or termination (1). Compared to other regions, the Caribbean region continues to have relatively high rates of adolescent pregnancy, with slow progress recorded in the past 30 years. During the 2010-2015 period, rates within the region ranged from 17 (Guadeloupe) to 101 (Dominican Republic) per 1,000 (15-19 year old) girls (2). Besides higher risks of life-threatening consequences during pregnancy and childbirth, adolescent pregnancy poses high costs for young mothers and their communities, mainly by perpetuating a cycle of poverty and social exclusion (2).

In a systematic review investigating risk and protective factors of adolescent pregnancy in low- and middle-income countries, Chung et al. (3) found, among many other factors, that older age, low socioeconomic status, sexual risk behaviors (such as transactional sex and multiple sexual partners), depressive symptoms, a history of sexual and physical abuse, low school attendance and low parental support increased the risk for adolescent pregnancy. Other factors, such as religion, contraceptive use, and substance use, showed mixed associations with adolescent pregnancy. This implies that the association between these risk and protective factors vary in different contexts, which needs to be taken into account when planning pregnancy prevention programs on a regional or national level (3).

Less is known about the risk and protective factors of adolescent pregnancy in Curaçao, a high-income Dutch Caribbean island. Adolescent pregnancy rates have fallen from 51 per 1,000 (15- to 19-year-old) girls in 1980-1984 to 37 per 1,000 girls in 2000-2005, but since then have failed to improve (2), between 175 and 200 girls have a child every year (4). Many adolescent pregnancies in Curaçao are unwanted resulting often (40-54%) in abortion (5). Adolescent pregnancy also seems to impact on long-term economic opportunities of young mothers in Curaçao: pregnant students have to temporarily leave school and more likely not to complete high school (6). To better tailor pregnancy prevention programmes aiming at reducing adolescent pregnancies, this study aimed to provide a better insight in the prevalence, risk and protective factors of adolescent pregnancy among adolescent girls in Curaçao.

OUR STUDY

Cross-sectional data from the 2015 Curaçao GSHS were analyzed (7). The study used a two-stage cluster sampling approach in order to generate representative data of all students enrolled in public secondary education, comparable to US Grades 1-6, in Curaçao. "At the first stage, 28 schools were selected with probability proportional to enrolment size, and at the second stage, 161 classes were randomly selected" (8). All students in selected classes were eligible to participate after ethical approval in accordance with the "WMA Declaration of Helsinki – Ethical Principles for Medical Research Involving Human Subjects" and other permissions were granted and informed consent was obtained from parents and children; the overall response rate was 83% (8).

MEASURES

The dataset from the self-administered GSHS questionnaire was used in this study (8). A description of the independent variables and their coding is depicted in appendix 1. Adolescent pregnancy was assessed with the question: "How many times have you been pregnant (for girls) or gotten someone pregnant (for boys)?" Answer options were 0 times, 1 time, 2 or more times, and "I don't know". Parental support (4 items) was categorized into 0-1 low, 2 medium and 3-4 high support. Psychological distress was defined as zero, single as one and multiple as 2-5 psychological distress, including the items loneliness, having no close friends, anxiety, suicidal ideation and suicide attempt.

Data analysis

Data analysis was conducted with STATA software version 15.0 (Stata Corporation, College Station, TX, USA), taking into account the complex study design. Unadjusted and adjusted multivariable logistic regression analyses were used to assess the associations between risk and protective factors with adolescent pregnancy: variables found significant in unadjusted analysis were subsequently included into the adjusted model. Cases with missing data were excluded from the analysis. P values <0.05 were considered significant.

FINDINGS

The sample included 1,508 school-going girls, with a median age of 16 years (interquartile range 3 years). Considering the prevalence of known risk factors for adolescent pregnancy, 6.1% of the female students had an early sexual debut, 16.6% had experience with multiple sexual partners,

Table 1. Characteristics of all (n = 1508) female students

Variable	Sample	Previously experienced pregnancy
	N (%)	%
All	1508 (100.0)	5.8
Age in years		
≤11-14	546 (31.4)	0.4
15-16	451 (32.6)	3.8
17-18 or more	507 (35.9)	12.0
Risk factors		
Experienced hunger	47 (3.2)	8.7
Early sexual debut (<14 years)	89 (6.1)	22.4
Multiple sexual partners	232 (16.6)	22.5
Transactional sex	21 (1.7)	28.6
History of forced sexual intercourse	121 (8.6)	15.1
Physical intimate partner violence victimization	137 (9.4)	10.3
Physical violence from parents	231 (15.8)	5.8
Current tobacco use	154 (10.8)	16.1
Heavy alcohol use	257 (18.7)	13.0
Current cannabis use	54 (4.1)	11.1
Cannot rely on any adult	259 (17.5)	8.9
Psychological distress		
0	870 (58.8)	3.9
1	309 (21.7)	5.7
2-5	274 (19.5)	9.1
Protective factors		
Religious or spiritual person	987 (70.7)	5.6
Parents provide necessities	1191 (84.0)	4.5
School attendance	1096 (73.8)	4.0
Peer support	705 (48.6)	5.3
Parental support		
Low	870 (26.6)	10.3
Medium	309 (25.6)	5.5
High	274 (47.8)	3.5
Lives with both parents	675 (45.0)	4.0
Ever talked about HIV/AIDS with parents	737 (52.4)	5.4

and 1.7% has had transactional sex. One in twelve (8.6%) female students had a history of forced sexual intercourse, 9.4% had experienced physical intimate partner violence victimization and 15.8% experienced violence

from their parents in the past 12 months. In terms of substance use, 10.8% were current tobacco users, 19.7% heavy alcohol users (≥2 drinks/day), and 4.1% were current cannabis users. One in five female students (19.5%) reported multiple psychological distress and 17.5% did not have any adult to rely on with their personal problems. Regarding the prevalence of known protective factors, 70.7% perceived themselves to be religious or spiritual, 84.0% received necessities from their parents, 73.8% attended school in the past month, 48.6% received mostly or always peer support, 47.8% had high parental support, 45.0% lived with both parents, and 52.4% had ever talked about HIV/AIDS with their parents. The prevalence of adolescent pregnancy was 5.8%, 1.4% of the female students reported to have been pregnant two or more times (see Table 1).

Contraceptive use

Table 2. Contraceptive use among female students who experienced pregnancy

Variable	Sample	Female students who experienced pregnancy
	N (%)	%
Preventive methods used		
Non-condom use at last sex	242 (17.6)	21.9
Non-birth control use at last sex	238 (16.8)	14.7
Main method used to prevent pregnancy		
Never had sex	849 (64.5)	0.0
Use of effective birth control, such as condoms, birth control pills, or an intra-uterine device to prevent pregnancy	264 (21.8)	16.4
Use of other methods of birth control, such as the withdrawal method or rhythm (safe time)	30 (2.3)	13.3
Morning after pill use	40 (3.2)	15.0
I do not try to prevent pregnancy, but if pregnancy occurs I would opt for abortion	18 (1.5)	38.9
Do not try to prevent pregnancy because I would like to have a child	22 (1.8)	9.1
Some other method	61 (4.9)	19.7

Among female students who had experienced pregnancy, 21.9% had not used a condom and 14.7% had not used birth control at last sex. As the main method to prevent pregnancy, 16.4% had used a reliable method of birth control, 13.3% other, less reliable, birth control methods, and 19.7% reported some other, unspecified, method. One in seven (15.0%) female students who had experienced pregnancy reported they used the morning after pill as the main method to prevent pregnancy. In addition, 38.9% of the female students did not try to prevent another pregnancy, as they would opt for abortion in the event of pregnancy, and 9.1% did not try to prevent pregnancy because they wanted to have a child (see Table 2).

Associations with adolescent pregnancy

In the unadjusted logistic regression analyses, sexual risk behaviors (early sexual debut, multiple sexual partners, and transactional sex), violent experiences (history of forced sexual intercourse and physical intimate partner violence victimization), substance use (current tobacco use, heavy alcohol use and current cannabis use), psychological distress and cannot rely on any adult when having personal problems were associated with adolescent pregnancy. Parental provision of necessities, school attendance and high parental support were protective for adolescent pregnancy. In the adjusted logistics regression analyses, having multiple sexual partners was positively and parental provision of necessities was negatively associated with adolescent pregnancy (see Table 3).

DISCUSSION

The study found that 5.8% of the school-going adolescent girls in Curaçao reported to have been pregnant. Among female students that had experienced pregnancy, only 16.4% used a reliable birth control method (condoms, the pill or an intra-uterine device), as a main method to prevent pregnancy, and 9.1% did not try to prevent pregnancy since they wanted to have a child. The remainder reported use of less reliable forms of birth control (withdrawal and the rhythm method, or some other unspecified method), the use of emergency contraception or to opt for abortion in the case of pregnancy, indicating that the majority of the previously pregnant girls remains at high risk for a recurrent unplanned pregnancy.

Table 3. Estimated association between risk and protective factors with adolescent pregnancy

Variable	UOR (95% CI)	AOR (95% CI)
Risk factors		
Experienced hunger	1.74 (0.48, 6.23)	---
Early sexual debut (<14 years)	6.48 (3.77, 11.15)***	1.88 (0.85, 4.17)
Multiple sexual partners	15.67 (9.72, 25.25)***	9.15 (4.63, 18.03)***
Transactional sex	6.07 (1.83, 20.11)**	1.32 (0.29, 6.09)
History of forced sexual intercourse	4.23 (2.37, 7.53)***	0.83 (0.34, 2.02)
Physical intimate partner violence victimization	2.35 (1.27, 4.35)**	1.17 (0.37, 3.64)
Physical violence from parents	1.19 (0.62, 2.30)	---
Current tobacco use	4.53 (2.64, 7.77)***	2.18 (0.96, 4.95)
Heavy alcohol use	3.51 (2.12, 5.82)***	1.66 (0.86, 3.21)
Current cannabis use	2.62 (1.14, 5.99)*	0.51 (0.18, 1.45)
Cannot rely on any adult	2.15 (1.29, 3.63)**	1.52 (0.86, 4.17)
Psychological distress		
0	1 (Reference)	1 (Reference)
1	1.36 (0.69, 2.71)	0.71 (0.26, 1.96)
2-5	2.39 (1.29, 4.44)**	0.94 (0.44, 1.98)
Protective factors		
Religious or spiritual person	0.96 (0.59, 1.58)	---
Parents provide necessities	0.35 (0.21, 0.59)***	0.43 (0.24, 0.76)**
School attendance	0.40 (0.25, 0.63)***	0.88 (0.49, 1.60)
Peer support	0.89 (0.56, 1.39)	---
Parental support		
Low	1 (Reference)	1 (Reference)
Medium	0.52 (0.24, 1.14)	1.10 (0.45, 2.63)
High	0.27 (0.15, 0.49)***	0.62 (0.27, 1.42)
Lives with both parents	0.58 (0.37, 0.90)*	1.07 (0.55, 2.12)
Ever talked about HIV/AIDS with parents	1/01 (0.62, 1.65)	---

UOR = Unadjusted Odds Ratio; AOR = Adjusted Odds Ratio; ***P < 0.001; **P < 0.01; *P < 0.05.

In line with other research findings (3), adolescent pregnancy in Curaçao was associated with various risk factors, including early sexual debut, multiple sexual partners, transactional sex, history of forced sexual intercourse, physical intimate partner violence victimization, substance use, cannot rely on any adult and psychological distress. Parents that provide necessities, school attendance, high parental support and living with both parents were protective from adolescent pregnancy. In contrast, factors such as experiencing hunger (as a proxy for socioeconomic background), experiencing physical violence from parents, thinking of oneself as a religious or spiritual person, peer support, and parental communication on HIV/AIDS (as a proxy for sex-education from parents) were not associated with adolescent pregnancy in Curaçao .

In adjusted logistic regression analysis, this study found a positive association between having multiple sexual partners and a negative association between the parental provision of necessities and adolescent pregnancy. A number of studies previously identified the influence of parent/child relationships on adolescents' sexual behaviour and hence, adolescent pregnancy risks. On the one hand, parental support is negatively related to adolescent pregnancy through reducing sexual intercourse and/or increasing contraceptive use (9). On the other hand, parental neglect for providing necessities makes adolescents prone to sexual exploitation by adults for providing basic needs, and unable to set the boundaries necessary to prevent pregnancy and sexually transmitted disease (10,11).

STUDY LIMITATIONS

The GSHS is limited to participants attending high schools in the public education system in Curaçao, which does not include out-off school adolescents and students in the private education system. Pregnant adolescents have to interrupt schooling in Curaçao, and will therefore not have been included in this survey, and students in the private sector may have fewer adolescent pregnancies due to better socio-economic circumstances. The questionnaire was administered by self-report, and therefore some of the responses may have been biased; sexual behavior, especially among females, may have been underreported. Some questions were not asked in this survey, such as accessibility to contraceptives, desirability of pregnancy, and outcomes of pregnancy, which should be included in future studies. The survey data were cross-sectional; no causal conclusions can be drawn from our results.

CONCLUSION

One in seventeen (5.8%) school-going girls in Curaçao reported to have been pregnant. The majority of these girls remain at high risk for a recurrent unplanned pregnancy. Knowledge of the identified risk factors, such as having multiple sexual partners and low parental provision of necessities, can assist in tailoring pregnancy prevention programmes.

APPENDIX 1. DESCRIPTION OF VARIABLES USED IN THIS STUDY

Variables	Question	Response options (Coding scheme)
	Sociodemographic factors	
Age	"How old are you?"	"11 years old or younger to 18 years old or older"
Sex	"What is your sex?"	"Male, Female"
	Outcome variable	
Adolescent pregnancy	How many times have you been pregnant or gotten someone pregnant?	"1 = 0 times to 3 = 2 or more times (coded 2-3 = 1 and 1 = 0)"
	Risk factors	
Non-birth control use at last sex	"The last time you had sexual intercourse, did you or your partner use any other method of birth control, such as withdrawal, rhythm (safe time), birth control pills, or any other method to prevent pregnancy?"	"Yes, No"

Variables	Question	Response options (Coding scheme)
	Risk factors	
Methods to prevent pregnancy	"What is the main method you use to prevent pregnancy?"	For example: "I use effective birth control, such as condoms, birth control pills, or an intra-uterine device to prevent pregnancy" (details Table 2)
Hunger	"During the past 30 days, how often did you go hungry because there was not enough food in your home?"	"1 = never to 5 = always (coded 1–3 = 0 and 4–5 = 1)"
Early sexual debut (<14 years)	"How old were you when you had sexual intercourse for the first time?"	"1 = never to 8 = 18 years old or older"
Two or more lifetime sexual partners	"During your life, with how many people have you had sexual intercourse?"	"1 = never to 7 = 6 or more people"
Transactional sex	"During your life, have you ever had sexual intercourse in exchange for something, such as a phone, jewellery, or money?"	"Yes, No"
Sexual violence victimization	"Have you ever been forced to have sexual intercourse when you did not want to?"	"Yes, No"
Physical partner violence victimization	"During the past 12 months, did your boyfriend or girlfriend ever hit, slap, or physically hurt you on purpose?"	"Yes, No"
Physical violence from parents	"During the past 12 months, did your parents or guardians ever hit, slap, or physically hurt you on purpose?"	"Yes, No"
Current tobacco use	"During the past 30 days, on how many days did you smoke cigarettes/use any tobacco products other than cigarettes, such as cigars, cigarillos, or electronic cigarettes?"	"1 = 0 days to 7 = All 30 days (coded 1 = 0 and 2-7 = 1)"
Heavy alcohol use (2 or more/day)	"During the past 30 days, on the days you drink alcohol, how many drinks did you usually drink per day?"	1 = Not drink in the past 30 days to 7 = 5 or more drinks (coded 1–3 = 0 and 4–7 = 1)
Current cannabis use	"During the past 30 days, how many times have you used marijuana (also called weed, pot, cannabis, ganja, or grass)?"	"1 = 0 days to 7 = All 30 days (coded 1 = 0 and 2-7 = 1)"

Appendix 1. (Continued)

Variables	Question	Response options (Coding scheme)
	Psychological distress	
Cannot rely on any adult	"How many adults can you rely on when you have personal problems?"	"1 = 0 to 4 = 3 or more (coded 1 = 1 and 2-4 = 0)"
No close friends	"How many close friends do you have?"	"1 = 0 to 4 = 3 or more (coded 1+ = 0, 0 = 1)"
Anxiety	"During the past 12 months, how often have you been so worried about something that you could not sleep at night?"	"1 = never to 5 = always (coded 1–3 = 0 and 4–5 = 1)"
Loneliness	"During the past 12 months, how often have you felt lonely?"	"1 = never to 5 = always (coded 1–3 = 0 and 4–5 = 1)"
Suicide ideation	"During the past 12 months, did you ever seriously consider attempting suicide?"	"Yes, No"
Suicide attempt	"During the past 12 months, how many times did you actually attempt suicide?"	"1 = 0 times to 5 = 6 or more times (coded 1 = 0 and 2–5 = 1)"
	Protective factors	
Religious or spiritual person	"Do you think of yourself as a religious or spiritual person?"	"Yes, No"
Provision of necessities	"During the past 30 days, how often did your parents or guardians provide for your necessities?"	"1 = never to 5 = always (coded 1–3 = 0 and 4–5 = 1)"
School attendance	"During the past 30 days, on how many days did you miss classes or school without permission?"	"1 = 0 days to 5 = 10 or more days (coded 1 = 0 and 2–5 = 1)"
Peer support	"During the past 30 days, how often were most of the students in your school kind and helpful?"-	"1 = never to 5 = always (coded 1–3 = 0 and 4–5 = 1)"
Parental supervision	"During the past 30 days, how often did your parents or guardians check to see if your homework was done?"	"1 = never to 5 = always (coded 1–3 = 0 and 4–5 = 1)"
Parental connectedness	"During the past 30 days, how often did your parents or guardians understand your problems and worries?"	"1 = never to 5 = always (coded 1–3 = 0 and 4–5 = 1)"
Parental bonding	"During the past 30 days, how often did your parents or guardians really know what you were doing with your free time?	"1 = never to 5 = always (coded 1–3 = 0 and 4–5 = 1)"

Variables	Question	Response options (Coding scheme)
	Protective factors	
Lives with both parents	"Which adult family members do you live with?"	"1 = both my mother and father to 5 = I do not live with any adult family members (coded 2-5 = 0 and 1 = 1)"
Ever talked about HIV/AIDS with parents	"Have you ever talked about HIV infection or AIDS with your parents or guardians?"	"Yes, No"

REFERENCES

[1] UNFPA. Adolescent pregnancy: A review of the evidence, 2013. URL: https://www.unfpa.org/sites/default/files/pub-pdf/ADOLESCENT%20 PREGNANCY_UNFPA.pdf.

[2] Pan American Health Organization (PAHO), United Nations Population Fund (UNPFA), United Nations Children's Fund (UNICEF). Accelerating progress toward the reduction of adolescent pregnancy in Latin America and the Caribbean. Report of a technical consultation. Washington: Pan American Health Organization; 2017. URL: https://lac.unfpa.org/sites/default/files/pub-pdf/Accelerating progress toward the reduction of adolescent pregnancy in LAC - FINAL.pdf.

[3] Chung HW, Kim EM, Lee JE. Comprehensive understanding of risk and protective factors related to adolescent pregnancy in low- and middle-income countries: A systematic review. J Adolesc 2018;69:180–8.

[4] Volksgezondheid Instituut Curaçao. Factsheet tienermoeders, 2015. URL: www.vic.cw.

[5] Boersma A, Alberts J, Bruijn J De, Meyboom BJ, Kleiverda G. Termination of pregnancy in Curaçao: need for improvement of sexual and reproductive healthcare. Glob J Health Sci 2012;4(3):30–8.

[6] Hellings E. Jong (&) Moeder. Willemstad, Curaçao, 2010. URL: http://www.faj.cw/index.php?topic = onderzoeksrapporten.

[7] World Health Organization (WHO). Global School-based Student Health Survey (GSHS). URL: http://www.who.int/chp/gshs/en/.

[8] Verstraeten S. The Curaçao Global School-based Student Health Survey (GSHS). Willemstad: Volksgezondheid Instituut Curaçao, 2015.

[9] Miller BC, Benson B, Galbraith KA. Family relationships and adolescent pregnancy risk: A research synthesis. Dev Rev 2001;21(1):1-38.

[10] Yakubu I, Salisu WJ. Determinants of adolescent pregnancy in sub-Saharan Africa: A systematic review. Reprod Health 2018;15(1):15. doi: 10.1186/s12978-018-0460-4.

[11] UNICEF. The situation of children and adolescents in Curaçao: key findings and recommendations, 2013. URL: https://www.unicef.nl/media/1371768/Curaçao_executive_summary__28english_29.pdf.

In: Adolescence in Curaçao
Editors: Soraya Verstraeten et al.
ISBN: 978-1-53617-522-6

Chapter 4

PREVALENCE AND CORRELATES OF SEXUAL VIOLENCE VICTIMIZATION AMONG A NATIONAL SAMPLE OF SCHOOL-GOING ADOLESCENTS IN CURAÇAO

Supa Pengpid[1,2,*], DrPH and Karl Peltzer[2], PhD
[1]ASEAN Institute for Health Development, Mahidol University, Salaya, Phutthamonthon, Nakhon Pathom, Thailand
[2]Department of Research Administration and Development, University of Limpopo, Turfloop, South Africa

ABSTRACT

In this chapter we assess sexual violence victimization among school-going adolescents in Curaçao. In the cross-sectional Curaçao "Global School-Based Student Health Survey (GSHS)" in 2015, 2,765 adolescents (median age 15 years) responded to questions on sexual

[*] ***Correspondence***: Professor Supa Pengpid, ASEAN Institute for Health Development, Mahidol University, 25/25 Phutthamonthon Road 4, Salaya, Phutthamonton, Nakhon Pathom 73170, Thailand. Email: supaprom@yahoo.com.

violence, sociodemographic factors, violence-related behaviours, substance use, sexual risk behaviour, psychological distress and protective factors. In all, 5.9% of students reported to have been forced to have sexual intercourse during their lifetime (=sexual violence victimization). The prevalence of sexual violence victimization was 2.9% among boys and 8.6% among girls. In adjusted logistic regression analyses among both sexes, female sex and multiple psychological distress were associated with sexual violence victimization. In addition, among both sexes and among girls, having been bullied, belonging to a violent group, physical violence victimization from parents, early sexual debut, multiple sexual partners and non-condom use at last sex were associated with sexual violence victimization. Almost one in ten girls reported sexual violence victimization and the knowledge of the identified risk factors can assist in tailoring prevention strategies.

INTRODUCTION

Sexual violence in childhood and adolescence is a major global public health problem, and has physical, sexual, reproductive and mental health consequences in the short and long term (1). Worldwide data suggest, "around 9% of girls and 3% of boys experienced attempted or completed forced intercourse (oral, vaginal, or anal)" (2). Findings from research in seven countries, the "lifetime prevalence of physically forced or pressured/coerced sexual intercourse among girls (0 to 18 years) ranged from a low of 1.5% in Cambodia to a high of 17.5% in Swaziland"(3); for "boys, this figure ranged from 0.2% in Cambodia to 7.6% in Haiti" (3). In national studies among adolescents in Brazil the lifetime sexual violence victimization was 4.0% (4) and in Ghana 18.6% (5) and United States 8.0% (6).

Risk factors for sexual violence victimization among female and/or male adolescents have included sociodemographic factors, violence-related behaviours, substance use, sexual risk behaviour, psychological distress and protective factors. Sociodemographic factors for sexual violence victimization include < 13 years old (4), increase in age (7), female (4, 8), black skin color (4) and working (4). Violence-related behaviours include being assaulted by family members (4), feeling insecure on the way to or at school (4), bullying victimization (4, 5), in a physical fight (9), physical dating violence victimization (9) and gun carrying (9).

Substance use risk factors for sexual violence victimization include tobacco use (4, 9), alcohol use, binge drinking and having been drunk (4, 8, 9), and having tried drugs (4). Sexual risk behaviours include having started sexual activity (4), having multiple recent sexual partners (9), and unprotected sex (4, 5). Psychological distress factors include having insomnia (4), feeling lonely (4), feeling sad/hopeless (9), depression (10), suicide ideation (9) and attempted suicide (9). Protective factors for sexual violence victimization may include having friends (4), living with parents (4), and supervision by relatives (4).

There is lack of information on the prevalence and correlates of sexual violence victimization among adolescents in some Caribbean countries, such as Curaçao. Knowing the prevalence and correlates of sexual violence victimizationr among adolescents in Curaçao will help in informing public health interventions aimed at preventing sexual violence. Consequently, the study aimed to assess the prevalence and correlates of sexual violence victimization among adolescents in Curaçao in 2015.

OUR STUDY

Cross-sectional data from the 2015 Curaçao GSHS were analyzed (11). The study used a two-stage cluster sample design to generate a representative sample of all students enrolled in public secondary education, comparable to US Grades 1-6, in Curaçao. "At the first stage, 28 schools were selected with probability proportional to enrolment size, and at the second stage, 161 classes were randomly selected" (12). All students in selected classes were eligible to participate after ethical approval **in accordance with the** *"WMA Declaration of Helsinki – Ethical Principles for Medical Research Involving Human Subjects"* and other permissions were granted and written informed consent was obtained from parents and children; the overall response rate was 83% (12).

Measures

The GSHS questionnaire applied to this analysis was used in this survey (see appendix 1) (13). Sexual violence victimization was assessed with the question "Have you ever been forced to have sexual intercourse when you did not want to?" The four parental support items were combined, resulting in 0-1 low, 2 medium and 3-4 high support. Psychological distress was defined as zero, single as one and multiple as 2-5 psychological distress (five items, including no close friends, loneliness, anxiety, suicidal ideation and suicide attempt).

Data analysis

Data analysis was conducted with "STATA software version 15.0 (Stata Corporation, College Station, TX, USA)," considering the complex sampling design. Unadjusted and adjusted logistic regression was used to assess the associations between independent variables (sociodemographic factors, violence-related behaviours, substance use, sexual risk behaviour, psychological distress and protective factors) and sexual violence victimization. Missing data were excluded from the analysis. P values <0.05 were considered significant.

FINDINGS

The sample consisted of 2,765 school-going adolescents, 51.1% female and 48.9% male, 3.8% had mostly or always experienced hunger in the past month, and 81.7% had parents or guardians that provided them mostly or always with necessities. In all, 5.9% of students reported to have been forced to have sexual intercourse during their lifetime (=sexual violence victimization). The prevalence of sexual violence victimization was 2.9% among boys and 8.6% among girls (see Table 1).

Table 1. Sample characteristics and sexual risk behaviour

Variable	Sample	Sexual violence victimization		
	Total	All	Male	Female
	N (%)	%	%	%
All	2765	5.9	2.9	8.6
	Sociodemographics			
Age in years				
≤11-14	1054 (32.8)	4.2	2.2	5.5
15-16	824 (32.7)	5.5	3.2	7.7
17-18 or more	877 (34.5)	7.8	2.9	12.1
Sex				
Female	1508 (51.1)			
Male	1230 (48.9)			
Parents provide necessities	2082 (81.7)	4.7	1.9	7.1
Experience hunger	102 (3.8)	13.3	7.2	14.4
Risk behaviour				
Current tobacco use	345 (13.2)	9.3	5.5	12.5
Heavy alcohol use	477 (19.0)	8.3	3.8	12.4
Current cannabis use	136 (5.7)	9.9	7.2	11.1
In physical fight	492 (17.9)	9.7	6.5	1.9
Physically attacked	394 (14.3)	10.5	5.1	14.2
Was bullied	683 (25.4)	10.0	4.3	14.9
Carried a weapon	363 (13.9)	8.3	4.2	13.3
Belongs to violent group	165 (6.1)	15.5	10.7	22.4
Physical violence from parents	417 (15.2)	12.7	6.1	18.0
Physical intimate partner violence victimization	282 (10.2)	9.2	5.4	13.1
Early sexual debut (<14 years)	230 (9.3)	18.1	8.0	35.3
Multiple sexual partners	480 (19.5)	14.3	5.6	1.8
Non-condom use at last sex	377 (15.1)	15.6	4.6	22.5
Transactional sex	60 (3.1)	17.9	9.6	36.7
Psychological distress				
0	1715 (65.1)	3.1	1.1	5.3
1	531 (20.5)	6.3	3.2	8.6
2-5	379 (14.4)	17.9	14.3	19.2
	Protective factors			
School attendance	1976 (73.4)	4.3	2.0	6.4
Peer support	1241 (47.6)	4.4	1.0	7.3
Lives with both parents	1325 (48.9)	3.9	3.1	4.8
Parental support				
Low	665 (27.2)	10.2	4.5	15.4
Medium	659 (26.7)	5.4	1.9	8.9
High	1167 (46.1)	3.3	1.6	4.9

Table 2. Associations with sexual violence victimization

Variable	Boys and girls		Girls
	UOR (95% CI)	AOR (95% CI)	AOR (95% CI)
	Sociodemographics		
Age in years			
≤11-14	1 (Reference)	1 (Reference)	1 (Reference)
15-16	1.32 (0.85, 2.04)	1.04 (0.55, 1.94)	1.15 (0.55, 2.44)
17-18 or more	1.93 (1.26, 2.96)**	1.51 (0.91, 2.48)	1.70 (0.89, 3.26)
Sex			
Female	1 (Reference)	1 (Reference)	---
Male	0.32 (0.21, 0.49)***	0.12 (0.06, 0.25)***	
Parents provide necessities	0.39 (0.25, 0.60)***	0.60 (0.30, 1.21)	0.73 (0.34, 1.56)
Experience hunger	2.60 (1.32, 5.14)***	1.46 (0.45, 4.74)	1.91 (0.58, 6.27)
Risk behaviour			
Current tobacco use	1.83 (1.07, 3.14)*	0.58 (0.26, 1.27)	0.81 (0.34, 1.94)
Heavy alcohol use	1.60 (1.08, 2.39)*	1.05 (0.58, 1.94)	0.80 (0.36, 1.77)
Current cannabis use	1.85 (0.97, 3.54)	---	---
In physical fight	1.98 (1.38, 2.83)***	0.96 (0.53, 1.74)	0.99 (0.47, 2.10)
Physically attacked	2.24 (1.44, 3.49)***	1.35 (0.78, 2.33)	1.48 (0.85, 2.58)
Was bullied	2.44 (1.70, 3.62)***	1.90 (1.10, 3.30)*	2.01 (1.09, 3.72)*
Carried a weapon	1.55 (0.83, 2.91)	---	---
Belongs to violent group	3.36 (2.07, 5.38)***	3.87 (1.64, 9.14)**	4.17 (1.54, 11.30)**
Physical violence from parents	2.92 (2.08, 4.08)***	1.79 (1.13, 2.85)*	2.24 (1.35, 3.73)**
Physical intimate partner violence victimization	1.77 (1.17, 2.68)**	0.72 (0.40, 1.29)	0.92 (0.48, 1.79)
Early sexual debut (<14 years)	4.56 (2.92, 7.11)***	2.86 (1.55 5.27)***	2.57 (1.33, 4.97)**
Multiple sexual partners	4.21 (3.20, 5.56)***	3.63 (2.09, 6.29)***	2.83 (1.53, 5.27)***
Non-condom use at last sex	4.29 (3.09, 5.95)***	2.31 (1.16, 4.58)*	2.31 (1.16, 4.58)*
Psychological distress			
0	1 (Reference)	1 (Reference)	1 (Reference)
1	2.12 (1.28, 3.50)**	1.15 (0.48, 2.78)	0.97 (0.37, 2.54)
2-5	6.79 (4.31, 10.68)***	2.93 (1.43, 5.98)**	1.96 (0.95, 4.04)
	Protective factors		
School attendance	0.37 (0.28, 0.50)***	0.82 (0.51, 1.34)	0.71 (0.44, 1.14)
Peer support	0.59 (0.38, 0.91)*	0.62 (0.38, 1.00)	0.70 (0.41, 1.18)
Lives with both parents	0.48 (0.33, 0.68)***	0.76 (0.48, 1.21)	0.67 (0.40, 1.13)
Parental support			
Low	1 (Reference)	1 (Reference)	1 (Reference)
Medium	0.50 (0.30, 0.82)**	0.99 (0.46, 2.15)	0.98 (0.42, 2.28)
High	0.30 (0.19, 0.47)***	0.91 (0.35, 2.34)	0.88 (0.27, 2.79)

UOR=Unadjusted odds ratio; AOR=Adjusted odds ratio; ***P<0.001; **P<0.01; *P<0.05.

Associations with sexual violence victimization

In adjusted logistic regression analyses among both sexes, female sex and multiple psychological distress were associated with sexual violence victimization. In addition, among both sexes and among girls, having been bullied, belonging to a violent group, physical violence victimization from parents, early sexual debut, multiple sexual partners and non-condom use at last sex were associated with sexual violence victimization (see Table 2).

DISCUSSION

The study found a prevalence of 5.9% (2.9% in males and 8.6% in females) sexual violence victimization in a nationally representative sample of in-school adolescents in Curaçao. These figures compare with worldwide estimates (3% in boys and 9% in girls) (2), is higher than in Brazil (4.0%) (4) and Cambodia (0.2% in boys and 1.5% in girls) (3), but is lower than in USA (8.0%) (6), Ghana (18.6%) (5), Swaziland (17.5% in girls) and Haiti (7.6% in boys) (3). Consistent with previous studies (4, 8), this study found that the prevalence of sexual violence victimization was significantly higher in female than male adolescents. The higher prevalence of sexual violence against females may be related to socio-cultural norms that support violence against girls and women (4, 5). Regarding the age of adolescents, previous studies (4, 7) found mixed results, while this study only found in unadjusted analysis that sexual violence victimization increased with age. Lower socioecomic status (experience of hunger and not being provided with necessities) was only in unadjusted analysis associated with sexual violence victimization. Economic inequality may increase the risk for sexual violence victimization (4).

In agreement with previous investigations (4, 5), this study found that parental physical violence victimization, bullying victimization and belonging to a violent group were associated with sexual violence victimization. While previous studies (9) found an association between in a physical fight, physical dating violence victimization, gun carrying and sexual violence victimization, this study found such associations only in unadjusted analysis for in physical fight and physical intimate partner violence victimization. While previous studies (4, 9), found an association between substance use and sexual violence victimization, this study only found in unadjusted analysis such an association with alcohol and tobacco use.

In consistence with previous research (5, 9), this investigation found that several sexual risk behaviours (early sexual debut, non-condom use at last sex, and multiple sexual partners) increased the odds for sexual violence victimization. This result shows that this vulnerable group is at increased risk for sexually transmitted infections and unwanted pregnancy (9). High psychological distress was among boys and girls but not among girls only associated with sexual violence victimization. Various previous studies (4, 9, 10) also found a link between different psychological distress indicators, such as loneliness, feeling sad or hopeless, depression, suicide ideation and suicide attempt and sexual violence victimization. This seems to show that adolescents with poorer mental health may be more vulnerable to circumstances that lead to sexual violence victimization (4). While previous studies (4) found different protective factors for sexual violence victimization, this study found this protective effect for school attendance, peer support, living with both parents and parental support only in unadjusted analysis.

Study limitations

The GSHS is limited to participants attending school, which does not include out-off school adolescents. The questionnaire administered was by self-report, and therefore some of the responses may have been biased, especially sexual violence, among both males and females, may have been underreported. The survey data were limited to a cross-sectional study design. The study did not assess the context, perpetrator and different time frames (lifetime, past 12 months) of sexual violence as well as health care seeking, which should be done in future studies.

CONCLUSION

Almost one in ten girls reported sexual violence victimization and the knowledge of the identified risk factors (violence related behaviour, sexual risk behaviour and psychological distress) can assist in tailoring prevention strategies. Further investigations are warrented to better understand the context of sexual violence in Curaçao.

APPENDIX 1. DESCRIPTION OF VARIABLES USED IN THIS STUDY

Variables	Question	Response options (Coding scheme)
	Sociodemographic factors	
Age	"How old are you?"	"11 years old or younger to 18 years old or older"
Sex	"What is your sex?"	"Male, Female"
Provision of necessities	"During the past 30 days, how often did your parents or guardians provide for your necessities?"	"1= never to 5= always (coded 1–3=0 and 4–5=1)"
Hunger	"During the past 30 days, how often did you go hungry because there was not enough food in your home?"	"1= never to 5= always (coded 1–3=0 and 4–5=1)"
	Outcome variable	
Sexual violence victimization	"Have you ever been forced to have sexual intercourse when you did not want to?"	"Yes, No"
	Risk behaviour	
Current tobacco use	"During the past 30 days, on how many days did you smoke cigarettes/use any tobacco products other than cigarettes, such as cigars, cigarillos, or electronic cigarettes?"	"1=0 days to 7=All 30 days (coded 1=0 and 2-7=1)"

Appendix 1. (Continued)

Variables	Question	Response options (Coding scheme)
	Risk behaviour	
Heavy alcohol use (2 or more/day)	"During the past 30 days, on the days you drink alcohol, how many drinks did you usually drink per day?"	1 = Not drink in the past 30 days to 7 = 5 or more drinks (coded 1–3 = 0 and 4–7 = 1)
Current cannabis use	"During the past 30 days, how many times have you used marijuana (also called weed, pot, cannabis, ganja, or grass)?"	"1=0 days to 7=All 30 days (coded 1=0 and 2-7=1)"
In a physical fight	"During the past 12 months, how many times were you in a physical fight?"	"1=0 times to 8=12 or more times (coded 1=0 and 2–8=1)"
Physically attacked	"During the past 12 months, how many times were you physically attacked?"	"1=0 times to 8=12 or more times (coded 1=0 and 2–8=1)"
Was bullied	"During the past 30 days, on how many days were you bullied?"	"1=0 days to 7=all 30 days (coded 1=0 and 2-7=1)"
Carried a weapon	"During the past 30 days, on how many days did you carry a weapon, such as a gun, knife, club, or brass knuckles?"	1=0 days to 5=6 or more days) (coded 1=0 and 2-6=1)
Belong to violent group	"Do you belong to any violent group?"	"Yes, No"
Physical violence from parents	"During the past 12 months, did your parents or guardians ever hit, slap, or physically hurt you on purpose?"	"Yes, No"
Physical partner violence victimization	"During the past 12 months, did your boyfriend or girlfriend ever hit, slap, or physically hurt you on purpose?"	"Yes, No"
Early sexual debut (<14 years)	"How old were you when you had sexual intercourse for the first time?"	"1=never to 8=18 years old or older"
Two or more lifetime sexual partners	"During your life, with how many people have you had sexual intercourse?"	"1=never to 7=6 or more people"
Non-condom use at last sex	"The last time you had sexual intercourse, did you or your partner use a condom or a rubber?"	"Yes, No"
Transactional sex	"During your life, have you ever had sexual intercourse in exchange for something, such as a phone, jewelry, or money?"	"Yes, No"
	Psychological distress	
No close friends	"How many close friends do you have?"	"1 = 0 to 4 = 3 or more (coded 1+=0, 0=1)"

Variables	Question	Response options (Coding scheme)
	Psychological distress	
Anxiety	"During the past 12 months, how often have you been so worried about something that you could not sleep at night?"	"1=never to 5=always (coded 1–3=0 and 4–5=1)"
Loneliness	"During the past 12 months, how often have you felt lonely?"	"1=never to 5=always (coded 1–3=0 and 4–5=1)"
Suicide ideation	"During the past 12 months, did you ever seriously consider attempting suicide?"	"Yes, No"
Suicide attempt	"During the past 12 months, how many times did you actually attempt suicide?"	"1=0 times to 5=6 or more times (coded 1=0 and 2–5=1)"
	Protective factors	
School attendance	"During the past 30 days, on how many days did you miss classes or school without permission?"	"1=0 days to 5= 10 or more days (coded 1=1 and 2–5=0)"
Peer support	"During the past 30 days, how often were most of the students in your school kind and helpful?"	"1=never to 5=always (coded 1–3=0 and 4–5=1)"
Lives with both parents	"Which adult family members do you live with?"	1=both my mother and father to 5=I do not live with any adult family members (coded 2-5=0 and 1=1)
Parental supervision	"During the past 30 days, how often did your parents or guardians check to see if your homework was done?"	"1=never to 5=always (coded 1–3=0 and 4–5=1)"
Parental connectedness	"During the past 30 days, how often did your parents or guardians understand your problems and worries?"	"1=never to 5=always (coded 1–3=0 and 4–5=1)"
Parental bonding	"During the past 30 days, how often did your parents or guardians really know what you were doing with your free time?	"1=never to 5=always (coded 1–3=0 and 4–5=1)"
Parental respect for privacy	"During the past 30 days, how often did your parents or guardians go through your things without your approval?"	"1=never to 5=always (coded 1–3=0 and 4–5=1)"

REFERENCES

[1] World Health Organization (WHO) Responding to children and adolescents who have been sexually abused: WHO clinical guidelines. Geneva, Switzerland: WHO, 2017.

[2] Barth J, Bermetz L, Heim E, Trelle S, Tonia T. The current prevalence of child sexual abuse worldwide: a systematic review and meta-analysis. Int J Public Health 2013;58(3):469–83. doi:10.1007/s00038-012-0426-1.

[3] Sumner S, Mercy JA, Saul J, Motsa-Nzuza N, Kwesigabo G, Buluma R et al. Prevalence of sexual violence against children and use of social services – seven countries, 2007-2013. MMWR 2015;64(21):565–9.

[4] Santos MJ, Mascarenhas MDM, Malta DC, Lima CM, Silva MMAD. Prevalence of sexual violence and associated factors among primary school students - Brazil, 2015. Cien Saude Colet 2019;24(2):535-44. doi: 10.1590/1413-81232018242.13112017.

[5] Ohene SA, Johnson K, Atunah-Jay S, Owusu A, Borowsky IW. Sexual and physical violence victimization among senior high school students in Ghana: Risk and protective factors. Soc Sci Med 2015;146:266-75.

[6] Howard DE, Wang MQ, Yan F. Prevalence and psychosocial correlates of forced sexual intercourse among U.S. high school adolescents. Adolescence 2007;42(168):629-43.

[7] Stark L, Seff I, Hoover A, Gordon R, Ligiero D, Massetti G. Sex and age effects in past-year experiences of violence amongst adolescents in five countries. PLoS One 2019;14(7):e0219073. doi: 10.1371/journal.pone.0219073. eCollection 2019.

[8] Dwyer T, Kulasingam S, Kamm KM, Chinunje D, Malamsha R, Mawji S, Kapinga R, Majinge C. Risk-taking behaviors and sexual violence among secondary school students in Tanzania. J Community Health 2019;44(4):749-55. doi: 10.1007/s10900-019-00673-2.

[9] Howard DE, Wang MQ. Psychosocial correlates of U.S. adolescents who report a history of forced sexual intercourse. J Adolesc Health 2005;36(5):372-9.

[10] Ngo QM, Veliz PT, Kusunoki Y, Stein SF, Boyd CJ. Adolescent sexual violence: Prevalence, adolescent risks, and violence characteristics. Prev Med 2018;116:68-74. doi: 10.1016/j.ypmed.2018.08.032.

[11] World Health Organization (WHO) Global School-based Student Health Survey (GSHS). 2015 Curacao. URL: https://www.who.int/ncds/surveillance/gshs/curacaodataset/en/.

[12] Verstraeten S. National report the Curaçao Global School-based Student Health Survey (GSHS) study 2015. URL: https://www.who.int/ncds/surveillance/gshs/Final_report_2015_GSHS_Curacao.pdf.

[13] World Health Organization (WHO) Global School-based Student Health Survey (GSHS). 2015 Curacao GSHS Questionnaire. URL: https://www.who.int/ncds/surveillance/gshs/2015_GSHS_Curacao_Questionnaire.pdf.

In: Adolescence in Curaçao
Editors: Soraya Verstraeten et al. ISBN: 978-1-53617-522-6

Chapter 5

EFFECTS OF FORCED SEXUAL INTERCOURSE ON HEALTH RISK BEHAVIOURS AND MENTAL HEALTH AMONG A NATIONAL SAMPLE OF IN-SCHOOL ADOLESCENTS IN CURAÇAO

Supa Pengpid[1,2,*], DrPH and Karl Peltzer[2], PhD
[1]ASEAN Institute for Health Development, Mahidol University, Salaya, Phutthamonthon, Nakhon Pathom, Thailand
[2]Department of Research Administration and Development, University of Limpopo, Turfloop, South Africa

ABSTRACT

In this chapter we investigate the effects of forced sexual intercourse among adolescents in Curaçao. In the cross-sectional Curaçao "Global School-Based Student Health Survey (GSHS)" in 2015, 2,765 adolescents (median age 15 years) responded to questions on forced

---

[*] ***Correspondence:*** Professor Supa Pengpid, ASEAN Institute for Health Development, Mahidol University, 25/25 Phutthamonthon Road 4, Salaya, Phutthamonton, Nakhon Pathom 73170, Thailand. Email: supaprom@yahoo.com.

sexual intercourse, sociodemographic factors, sexual risk behaviour, violence related behaviour, mental health and substance use. The lifetime prevalence for history of forced sexual intercourse was 5.9%, 2.9% among boys and 8.6% among girls. In adjusted logistic regression analyses among both sexes and among girls forced sexual intercourse increased the odds for sexual risk behaviours (early sexual debut, multiple sexual partners, transactional sex, non-condom use at last sex, non-birth control use at last sex and adolescent pregnancy), violence related behaviour (in a physical fight, physically attacked, belonging to a violent group, was bulled and having experienced physical violence from parents), poor mental health (anxiety, loneliness, suicide ideation, plan and attempt) and substance use (ever used methamphetamine, cocaine or XTC). In addition, among boys, forced sexual intercourse increased the odds for having no close friends and current cannabis use. A lifetime history of forced sexual intercourse was associated with sexual risk behaviours, including pregnancy, violence related behaviours, poor mental health and substance use. Interventions programmes targeting victimized adolescents should address linked health risk behaviours identified.

INTRODUCTION

According to UNICEF (1):

> "Sexual violence such as forced sexual intercourse experienced as a child can have a profound impact on core aspects of emotional, behavioral and physical health and social development throughout life. Sexual violence can also result in immediate and chronic physical and psychological consequences as wide ranging as heart disease to symptoms of posttraumatic stress disorder, depression and attempted or completed suicide. Sexual violence is also associated with increased risk of sexual and reproductive health problems, including unintended pregnancy, HIV and other sexually transmitted infections."

Various studies have identified that a history of forced sexual intercourse among adolescents is associated with sexual risk behaviours, violence related behaviours, poor mental health and substance use. Sexual risk behaviours may include early sexual debut (2), multiple sexual partners

(2), unprotected sex (2, 3) and unwanted pregnancy (4). Violence related behaviour may include in a physical fight (2), physical violence (3), physical dating violence (5), carried a weapon (2), bullied (2), and school truancy (2). Poor mental health because of forced sexual intercourse may include mental distress (3), depressed symptoms (4), suicide ideation (3-5), hurting oneself (3), and difficulty sleeping (4). Several studies found that a history of forced sexual intercourse among adolescents increased the odds for substance use (2, 5), alcohol use (2, 4), tobacco use (2), cannabis use (2), and other drugs such as methamethamine (2).

In order to better understand the context of the negative effects of sexual violence in a Caribbean context, this study aimed to investigate the effects of forced sexual intercourse among a national sample of in-school adolescents in Curaçao.

OUR STUDY

Cross-sectional data from the 2015 Curaçao GSHS were analyzed (6). The study used a two-stage cluster sample design to produce data representative of all students enrolled in public secondary education, comparable to US Grades 1-6, in Curaçao. "At the first stage, 28 schools were selected with probability proportional to enrolment size, and at the second stage, 161 classes were randomly selected" (7). All students in selected classes were eligible to participate after ethical approval *in accordance with the "WMA Declaration of Helsinki – Ethical Principles for Medical Research Involving Human Subjects"* and other permissions were granted and written informed consent was obtained from parents and children; the overall response rate was 83% (7).

Measures

The GSHS questionnaire applied to this analysis was used in this survey (see Appendix 1) (8). The four items on parental support were combined into 0-1 low, 2 medium and 3-4 high support. Short sleep was defined as less than the normal or recommended sleep duration of "9-11 hours for 6-13 year-old children, 8-10 hours for 14-17 year-olds and 7-9 hours for 18-25 year-olds" (9).

Data analysis

Data analysis was conducted with "STATA software version 15.0 (Stata Corporation, College Station, TX, USA)", considering the complex study approach. Multivariable logistic regression was used to assess the associations between forced sexual intercourse, relevant confounders (age, sex, hunger, parental provision of necessities, living status, peer and parental support) and dependent variables (19 health risk behaviours and seven poor mental health indicators). Missing data were excluded from the analysis. P values <0.05 were considered significant.

FINDINGS

The sample consisted of 2,765 school-going adolescents, 51.1% female and 48.9% male, 3.8% had mostly or always experienced hunger in the past month, 81.7% had parents or guardians that provided them mostly or always with necessities, 47.6% had peer support, 48.9% lived with both parents and 46.1% had high parental support. In all, 5.9% of students reported to have been forced to have sexual intercourse during their lifetime. The prevalence of forced sexual intercourse was 2.9% among boys and 8.6% among girls.

Table 1. Adjusted associations between forced sexual intercourse and health risk behaviours

Variable	All	Male	Female
	AOR (95% CI)[1]	AOR (95% CI)[1]	AOR (95% CI)[1]
Sexual risk behaviour			
Early sexual debut (<14 years) (9.3%)	5.47 (3.45, 8.68)***	6.20 (2.39, 16.06)***	5.44 (3.27, 9.06)***
Multiple sexual partners (19.5%)	5.01 (3.62, 6.93)***	4.85 (1.36, 17.25)*	5.60 (3.54, 8.88)***
Transactional sex (3.1%)	3.65 (1.42, 9.33)**	2.47 (0.32, 18.98)	5.06 (1.69, 15.12)**
Non-condom use at last sex (15.1%)	3.11 (1.97, 4.94)***	1.07 (0.26, 4.43)	3.99 (2.38, 6.67)***
Non-birth control use at last sex (20.3%)	3.65 (1.42, 5.31)***	2.97 (0.80, 11.13)	3.48 (2.01, 6.02)***
Adolescent pregnancy (4.7%)	2.18 (1.26, 3.78)**	1.66 (0.30, 9.01)	2.34 (1.24, 4.41)**
Violence related behaviour			
In physical fight (17.9%)	2.30 (1.55, 3.40)***	3.43 (1.21, 9.64)*	1.89 (1.23, 2.93)**
Physically attacked (14.3)	1.89 (1.18, 3.04)**	1.69 (0.58, 4.92)	1.92 (1.14, 3.22)*
Carried a weapon (13.9%)	1.25 (0.62, 2.51)	1.07 (0.39, 2.96)	1.28 (0.61, 2.72)
Belong to violent group (6.1%)	4.06 (2.12, 7.43)***	5.32 (1.49, 19.01)*	3.35 (1.50, 7.47)**
Was bullied (25.4%)	2.26 (1.50, 3.41)***	1.54 (0.62, 3.82)	2.58 (1.60, 4.17)***
Physical partner violence victimization (10.2%)	1.34 (0.85, 2.13)	0.72 (0.16, 3.17)	1.53 (0.96, 2.45)
Physical violence from parents (15.2%)	2.71 (1.92, 3.83)***	2.58 (1.09, 6.15)*	2.65 (1.81, 3.88)***
School truancy (26.6%)	2.02 (1.43, 2.85)***	2.45 (1.02, 5.86)*	1.95 (1.32, 2.88)***
Mental health			
No close friends	1.40 (0.83, 2.37)	2.93 (1.04, 8.24)*	1.11 (0.66, 1.86)
Anxiety (11.4%)	2.93 (1.80, 4.78)***	4.77 (1.00, 22.79)	2.62 (1.54, 4.45)***
Loneliness (15.5%)	2.20 (1.38, 3.49)***	3.38 (1.32, 8.66)*	2.13 (1.23, 3.70)**
Suicide ideation (11.3%)	3.03 (2.02, 4.53)***	4.86 (1.25, 17.59)*	2.76 (1.74, 4.36)***
Suicide plan (9.1%)	3.11 (1.91, 5.06)***	4.12 (1.13, 15.02)*	2.91 (1.86, 4.56)***

Table 1. (Continued)

Variable	All	Male	Female
	AOR (95% CI)[1]	AOR (95% CI)[1]	AOR (95% CI)[1]
Suicide attempt (10.8%)	2.63 (1.64, 4.23)***	2.87 (0.88, 9.32)	2.61 (1.58, 4.31)***
Short sleep (63.3%)	0.75 (0.48, 1.18)	0.54 (0.16, 1.85)	0.84 (0.54, 1.31)
Substance use			
Current alcohol use (40.8%)	1.24 (0.82, 1.86)	1.85 (0.68, 5.03)	1.15 (0.72, 1.85)
Current tobacco use (13.2%)	1.33 (0.76, 2.35)	1.25 (0.38, 4.14)	1.35 (0.70, 2.57)
Current cannabis use (5.7%)	1.55 (0.72, 3.34)	3.73 (1.09, 12.73)*	1.02 (0.39, 2.68)
Used methamphetamine, cocaine, or XTC one or more times (1.3%)	5.29 (2.02, 13.88)***	16.18 (3.41, 76.83)***	3.40 (1.15, 10.04)*

AOR = Adjusted Odds Ratio; ***P < 0.001; **P < 0.01; *P < 0.05;

[1]Adjusted for age, sex, hunger, parental provision of necessities, living status (with both parents), peer and parental support.

Associations between forced sexual intercourse and health risk behaviour

In adjusted logistic regression analyses among both sexes and among girls forced sexual intercourse increased the odds for sexual risk behaviours (early sexual debut, multiple sexual partners, transactional sex, non-condom use at last sex, non-birth control use at last sex and adolescent pregnancy), violence related behaviour (in a physical fight, physically attacked, belonong to a violent group, was bulled and having experienced physical violence from parents), poor mental health (anxiety, loneliness, suicide ideation, plan and attempt) and substance use (ever used methamphetamine, cocaine or XTC). In addition, among boys, forced sexual intercourse was associated with having no close friends and current cannabis use (see Table 1).

DISCUSSION

In agreement with a number of previous studies (1-5), this study found among both boys and girls and among girls only that having experienced forced sexual intercourse increased the likelihood of seven sexual risk behaviours, six of eight violence related behaviours, five of seven poor mental health indicators and one of four substance use types. These findings replicate earlier results showing the wide range of possible effects of forced sexual intercourse on various health risk behaviours and poor mental indicators (5).

Possible mechanisms to explain the effects of forced sexual intercourse on sexual risk behaviours may stem from a "neurobiological dysregulation" affecting psychosocial and cognitive development in the form of feeling powerless, low self-esteem and depression leading sexual risk behaviours, reducing one's ability to negotiate protective barrier or contraceptive use and to engage in a secure and maintain a relationship (10). Likewise, the sexual violence experience may enact a vulnerability to other violence related behaviours such as physical violence victimization from parents, in a physical fight, physically attacked, having been bullied and belonging to a violent group. The experience of poor mental health may trigger negative copying strategies, such as self-medication with drugs or violence related behaviour.

Unlike a previous study (5), this study did not find an association between forced sexual intercourse and physical partner violence victimization. The study also failed to find an association between forced sexual intercourse and alcohol and tobacco use, as found in some previous studies (2,4), and cannabis use only among boys, as found previously (2). Secondary prevention is indicated to prevent or mitigate the negative health consequences of sexual violence in this population.

Study limitations

The GSHS is limited to participants attending school, which does not include out-off school adolescents. The questionnaire administered was by self-report, and therefore some of the responses may have been biased; forced sexual intercourse may have been underreported among both boys and girls. Forced sexual intercourse was only assessed with one question, and future studies should consider several questions and provide definitions of terminology, such as "sexual intercourse" or "forced" used. The survey data were limited to cross-sectional design.

Conclusion

A lifetime history of forced sexual intercourse was associated with sexual risk behaviours, including pregnancy, violence related behaviours, poor mental health and substance use. Interventions programmes targeting victimized adolescents should address linked health risk behaviours identified in Curaçao.

APPENDIX 1. DESCRIPTION OF VARIABLES USED IN THIS STUDY

Variables	Question	Response options (Coding scheme)
	Sociodemographic and protective factors	
Age	"How old are you?"	"11 years old or younger to 18 years old or older"
Sex	"What is your sex?"	"Male, Female"
Provision of necessities	"During the past 30 days, how often did your parents or guardians provide for your necessities?"	"1 = never to 5 = always (coded 1–3 = 0 and 4–5 = 1)"
Hunger	"During the past 30 days, how often did you go hungry because there was not enough food in your home?"	"1 = never to 5 = always (coded 1–3 = 0 and 4–5 = 1)"
Peer support	"During the past 30 days, how often were most of the students in your school kind and helpful?"	"1 = never to 5 = always (coded 1–3 = 0 and 4–5 = 1)"
Lives with both parents	"Which adult family members do you live with?"	1 = both my mother and father to 5 = I do not live with any adult family members (coded 2-5 = 0 and 1 = 1)
Parental supervision	"During the past 30 days, how often did your parents or guardians check to see if your homework was done?"	"1 = never to 5 = always (coded 1–3 = 0 and 4–5 = 1)"
Parental connectedness	"During the past 30 days, how often did your parents or guardians understand your problems and worries?"	"1 = never to 5 = always (coded 1–3 = 0 and 4–5 = 1)"
Parental bonding	"During the past 30 days, how often did your parents or guardians really know what you were doing with your free time?	"1 = never to 5 = always (coded 1–3 = 0 and 4–5 = 1)"
Parental respect for privacy	"During the past 30 days, how often did your parents or guardians go through your things without your approval?"	"1 = never to 5 = always (coded 1–3 = 0 and 4–5 = 1)"
	Predictor variable	
Sexual violence victimization	"Have you ever been forced to have sexual intercourse when you did not want to?"	"Yes, No"

Appendix 1. (Continued)

Variables	Question	Response options (Coding scheme)
	Outcome variables	
Early sexual debut (<14 years)	"How old were you when you had sexual intercourse for the first time?"	"1 = never to 8 = 18 years old or older"
Two or more lifetime sexual partners	"During your life, with how many people have you had sexual intercourse?"	"1 = never to 7 = 6 or more people"
Transactional sex	"During your life, have you ever had sexual intercourse in exchange for something, such as a phone, jewelry, or money?"	"Yes, No"
Non-condom use at last sex	"The last time you had sexual intercourse, did you or your partner use a condom or a rubber?"	"Yes, No"
Non-birth control use at last sex	"The last time you had sexual intercourse, did you or your partner use any other method of birth control, such as withdrawal, rhythm (safe time), birth control pills, or any other method to prevent pregnancy?"	"Yes, No"
Adolescent pregnancy	How many times have you been pregnant or gotten someone pregnant?	"1 = 0 times to 3 = 2 or more times (coded 2-3 = 1 and 1 = 0)"
In a physical fight	"During the past 12 months, how many times were you in a physical fight?"	"1 = 0 times to 8 = 12 or more times (coded 1 = 0 and 2–8 = 1)"
Physically attacked	"During the past 12 months, how many times were you physically attacked?"	1 = 0 times to 8 = 12 or more times (coded 1 = 0 and 2–8 = 1)
Carried a weapon	"During the past 30 days, on how many days did you carry a weapon, such as a gun, knife, club, or brass knuckles?"	1 = 0 days to 5 = 6 or more days) (coded 1 = 0 and 2-6 = 1)
Belong to violent group	"Do you belong to any violent group?"	"Yes, No"
Was bullied	"During the past 30 days, on how many days were you bullied?"	"1 = 0 days to 7 = all 30 days (coded 1 = 0 and 2-7 = 1)"
Physical partner violence victimization	"During the past 12 months, did your boyfriend or girlfriend ever hit, slap, or physically hurt you on purpose?"	"Yes, No"

Variables	Question	Response options (Coding scheme)
Outcome variables		
Physical violence from parents	"During the past 12 months, did your parents or guardians ever hit, slap, or physically hurt you on purpose?"	"Yes, No"
No close friends	"How many close friends do you have?"	"1 = 0 to 4 = 3 or more (coded 1+ = 0, 0 = 1)"
Anxiety	"During the past 12 months, how often have you been so worried about something that you could not sleep at night?"	"1 = never to 5 = always (coded 1–3 = 0 and 4–5 = 1)"
Loneliness	"During the past 12 months, how often have you felt lonely?"	"1 = never to 5 = always (coded 1–3 = 0 and 4–5 = 1)"
Suicide ideation	"During the past 12 months, did you ever seriously consider attempting suicide?"	"Yes, No"
Suicide plan	"During the past 12 months, did you make a plan about how you would attempt suicide?"	"Yes, No"
Suicide attempt	"During the past 12 months, how many times did you actually attempt suicide?"	"1 = 0 times to 5 = 6 or more times (coded 1 = 0 and 2–5 = 1)"
Sleep duration	"On an average school night, how many hours of sleep do you get?"	"1 = 4 or less hours to 7 = 10 or more hours)"
Current alcohol use	"During the past 30 days, on how many days did you have at least one drink containing alcohol?"	"1 = 0 days to 7 = All 30 days (coded 1 = 0 and 2-7 = 1)"
Current tobacco use	"During the past 30 days, on how many days did you smoke cigarettes/use any tobacco products other than cigarettes, such as cigars, cigarillos, or electronic cigarettes?"	"1 = 0 days to 7 = All 30 days (coded 1 = 0 and 2-7 = 1)"
Current cannabis use	"During the past 30 days, how many times have you used marijuana (also called weed, pot, cannabis, ganja, or grass)?"	"1 = 0 days to 7 = All 30 days (coded 1 = 0 and 2-7 = 1)"
Lifetime methamphetamine, etc. use	"During your life, how many times have you used methamphetamine, cocaine, or XTC (also called speed, base, rock, crack, and uppers)?"	"1 = 0 times to 5 = 20 or more times (coded 1 = 0 and 2-5 = 1)"

REFERENCES

[1] UNICEF. Together for girls: Sexual violence fact Sheet, 2012. URL: https://www.unicef.org/protection/files/Together_for_Girls_Sexual_Violence_Fact_Sheet_July_2012.pdf.

[2] Lowry R, Robin L, Kann L. Effect of forced sexual intercourse on asociations between sexual debut and other health risk behaviors among US high school students. J Sch Health 2017;87(6):435-47. doi: 10.1111/josh.12512.

[3] Nguyen KH, Padilla M, Villaveces A, Patel P, Atuchukwu V, Onotu D, et al. Coerced and forced sexual initiation and its association with negative health outcomes among youth: Results from the Nigeria, Uganda, and Zambia Violence Against Children Surveys. Child Abuse Negl 2019;96:104074. doi: 10.1016/j.chiabu.2019.104074.

[4] Reza A, Breiding MJ, Gulaid J, Mercy JA, Blanton C, Mthethwa Z, et al. Sexual violence and its health consequences for female children in Swaziland: A cluster survey study. Lancet 2009;373(9679):1966-72. doi: 10.1016/S0140-6736(09)60247-6.

[5] Basile KC, Black MC, Simon TR, Arias I, Brener ND, Saltzman LE. The association between self-reported lifetime history of forced sexual intercourse and recent health-risk behaviors: findings from the 2003 National Youth Risk Behavior Survey. J Adolesc Health 2006;39(5):752.e1-7.

[6] World Health Organization (WHO) Global School-based Student Health Survey (GSHS). 2015 Curacao. URL: https://www.who.int/ncds/surveillance/gshs/curacaodataset/en/.

[7] Verstraeten S. National report the Curaçao Global School-based Student Health Survey (GSHS) study 2015. URL: https://www.who.int/ncds/surveillance/gshs/Final_report_2015_GSHS_Curacao.pdf.

[8] World Health Organization (WHO) Global School-based Student Health Survey (GSHS). 2015 Curacao GSHS Questionnaire. URL: https://www.who.int/ncds/surveillance/gshs/2015_GSHS_Curacao_Questionnaire.pdf.

[9] National sleep foundation. National sleep foundation recommends new sleep times, 2019. URL: https://www.sleepfoundation.org/press-release/national-sleep-foundation-recommends-new-sleep-times/page/0/1.

[10] Homma Y, Wang N, Saewyc E, Kishor N. The relationship between sexual abuse and risky sexual behaviour among adolescent boys: A meta-analysis. J Adolesc Health 2012;51(1):18-24. doi: 10.1016/j.jadohealth.2011.12.032.

In: Adolescence in Curaçao
Editors: Soraya Verstraeten et al.
ISBN: 978-1-53617-522-6

Chapter 6

PREVALENCE AND PREDICTORS OF PAST 12 MONTHS PHYSICAL INTIMATE PARTNER VIOLENCE VICTIMIZATION AMONG A NATIONAL SAMPLE OF SCHOOL-GOING ADOLESCENTS IN CURAÇAO

Supa Pengpid*[1,2,*]*, DrPH, Karl Peltzer*[2]*, PhD and Soraya Verstraeten*[3]*, MSc

[1]ASEAN Institute for Health Development, Mahidol University, Salaya, Phutthamonthon, Nakhon Pathom, Thailand
[2]Department of Research Administration and Development, University of Limpopo, Turfloop, South Africa
[3]Institute for Public Health (Volksgezondheid Instituut Curaçao), Ministry of Public Health, Environment and Nature, Willemstad, Curaçao

[*] ***Correspondence***: Professor Supa Pengpid, ASEAN Institute for Health Development, Mahidol University, 25/25 Phutthamonthon Road 4, Salaya, Phutthamonton, Nakhon Pathom 73170, Thailand. Email: supaprom@yahoo.com.

ABSTRACT

In the cross-sectional Curaçao "Global School-Based Student Health Survey" (GSHS) in 2015, 2,765 adolescents (median age 15 years) responded to questions on sociodemographic factors, risk behaviours, psychological distress and protective factors. The prevalence of past 12-month physical intimate partner violence (IPV) victimization was 10.5% (11.6% among boys and 9.4% among girls). In the adjusted logistic regression analyses, parental provision of necessities was negatively and early sexual debut was positively associated with recent physical IPV victimization between both sexes. In addition, among boys, belonging to a violent group, and among girls, being bullied and non-condom use at last sex were positively and medium parental support was negatively associated with recent physical IPV victimization. More than one in ten school-going adolescents had been victim of physical IPV. Interventions to prevent physical IPV victimization in this population may include multiple levels, including school-based, community-based and parenting interventions.

INTRODUCTION

"Internationally, population-based studies of dating violence are few, but limited evidence suggests that this affects a substantial proportion of youth" (1). Several studies among American adolescents report that physical intimate partner violence (IPV) victimization ranges from 7.8% to 13.5% in both genders, with similar rates for boys (7.6%-12.9%) and girls (8%-14.4%) (2-6). In two studies in South Africa, the prevalence of physical IPV victimization among adolescents was 21.1% for boys and 12.4% to 39% for girls (7, 8). Less is known about the prevalence and correlates of IPV among adolescents in the Caribbean region, Curaçao in particular. Among Curaçaoan adults, the lifetime prevalence of domestic violence was 25% among men and 38% among women (9); some of the risk factors included female sex, young age, and a history of domestic violence victimization during childhood (9).

Risk factors of physical IPV victimization among adolescents may include sociodemographic factors, substance use, violence related behaviour, sexual risk behaviour, psychological distress and protective factors. Sociodemographic risk factors for physical IPV victimization among adolescents (boys and/or girls) may include older age (4, 10), being male (7), and being female (11). Substance use risk factors may include alcohol use (10), binge drinking (5, 12) and illicit drug use (10).

Violence related behaviour associated with physical IPV victimization among adolescent boys and/or girls include physical fighting (3), gun carrying (3, 5), sexual violence victimization, sexual abuse (4), ever been forced to have sex (4), gang membership (13), bullying (12), intra-familial violence (10, 14), being a victim of violence by an adult household member (14). Sexual risk behaviours may include being sexually active or ever had sex (4, 15), not using a condom (3, 16), and having multiple sexual partners (3, 10).

Psychological distress, such as being sad or hopeless (3), suicidality (4), and suicidal ideation (5) have been associated with physical IPV victimization among adolescent boys and /or girls. Factors that may be protective from physical IPV victimization among adolescents may include high-perceived care by teachers and friends (14), high-perceived care by parents (12, 14), parental monitoring (2) and religious service attendance (2).

Given the lack of information on the prevalence and predictors of physical IPV victimization among adolescents in the Caribbean region, this study presents the results from Curaçao. Knowing the prevalence and predictors of physical IPV victimization can inform public health interventions aimed at the prevention of IPV. Consequently, this study aimed to assess the prevalence and predictors of physical IPV victimization among adolescents in Curaçao in 2015.

OUR STUDY

Cross-sectional data from the 2015 Curaçao GSHS were analyzed (17). The study used a two-stage cluster sampling approach to generate representative data of all students enrolled in public secondary education, comparable to US Grades 1-6, in Curaçao. "At the first stage, 28 schools were selected with probability proportional to enrolment size, and at the second stage, 161 classes were randomly selected" (18). All students in selected classes were eligible to participate after ethical approval in accordance with the "WMA Declaration of Helsinki – Ethical Principles for Medical Research Involving Human Subjects" and other permissions were granted and written informed consent was obtained from parents and children; the overall response rate was 83% (18).

Measures

The dataset from the self-administered GSHS questionnaire was utilized in this study. A description of the independent variables and their coding is depicted in Appendix 1 (19). Past 12-month physical IPV victimization was assessed with the question: "During the past 12 months, did your boyfriend or girlfriend ever hit, slap, or physically hurt you on purpose (Yes, No)?" Parental support (four items) was categorized into 0-1 low, 2 medium and 3-4 high support. Psychological distress was defined as zero, single as one and multiple as 2-5 psychological distress, including the items loneliness, having no close friends, anxiety, suicidal ideation and suicide attempt.

Data analysis

Data analysis was conducted with "STATA software version 15.0 (Stata Corporation, College Station, TX, USA)," considering the complex study approach. Frequency tabulations were used in describing the sample. Logistic regression was used to assess the associations between independent variables (sociodemographic factors, risk behaviour, psychological distress, and protective factors) and past 12-month physical IPV victimization. Variables found significant at $P<0.05$ level in the bivariate analyses were included in the multivariable model, overall, and for boys and girls separately. P values of <0.05 were considered significant.

FINDINGS

The sample consisted of 2,765 school-going adolescents, 51.1% female and 48.9% male, 3.8% had experienced hunger in the past 30 days, and 81.7% had parents or guardians that provided them mostly or always with necessities. More than two thirds (69.0%) of the students perceived themselves to be a religious or spiritual person, 73.4% did not skip school without permission in the past month, 47.6% received peer support in the past month and 46.1% scored high on parental support. The prevalence of various risk behaviours and psychological distress is described in Table 1. Overall, the prevalence of past 12-month physical IPV victimization was 10.5%, 11.6% among boys and 9.4% among girls (see Table 1).

Table 1. Sample and physical partner violence victimization characteristics

Variable	Sample	Physical partner violence victimization		
	Total	All	Male	Female
	N (%)	%	%	%
All	2765	10.5	11.6	9.4
Sociodemographics				
Age in years				
≤11-14	1054 (32.8)	9.0	11.4	6.4
15-16	824 (32.7)	10.2	10.0	10.5
17-18 or more	877 (34.5)	12.2	13.3	11.1
Sex				
Female	1508 (51.1)			
Male	1230 (48.9)			
Parents provide necessities	2082 (81.7)	9.0	9.4	8.5
Experience hunger	102 (3.8)	17.4	16.4	17.8
Risk behaviour				
Current tobacco use	345 (13.2)	18.0	20.1	14.8
Heavy alcohol use	477 (19.0)	12.1	12.7	15.1
Current cannabis use	136 (5.7)	18.6	22.6	13.6
In physical fight	492 (17.9)	13.9	14.2	13.4

Table 1. (Continued)

Variable	Sample	Physical partner violence victimization		
	Total	All	Male	Female
	N (%)	%	%	%
Physically attacked	394 (14.3)	12.8	12.9	12.5
Was bullied	683 (25.4)	12.4	10.4	14.3
Carried a weapon	363 (13.9)	17.8	17.4	18.4
Belongs to violent group	165 (6.1)	23.5	27.7	16.9
Physical violence from parents	417 (15.2)	10.4	13.3	8.1
Sexual violence victimization	159 (5.9)	16.6	23.0	14.0
Early sexual debut (<14 years)	230 (9.3)	19.5	19.5	18.9
Multiple sexual partners	480 (19.5)	17.0	17.6	16.4
Non-condom use at last sex	377 (15.1)	17.6	17.6	17.5
Psychological distress				
0	1715 (65.1)	9.4	10.9	7.7
1	531 (20.5)	10.6	13.6	7.8
2-5	379 (14.4)	14.3	11.3	15.7
Protective factors				
School attendance	1976 (73.4)	8.9	9.7	8.1
Religious person	1717 (69.0)	9.7	9.7	9.6
Peer support	1241 (47.6)	9.0	10.4	7.8
Lives with both parents	1325 (48.9)	10.4	9.6	11.1
Parental support				
Low	665 (27.2)	14.2	14.1	14.0
Medium	659 (26.7)	8.4	10.6	6.0
High	1167 (46.1)	9.2	9.8	8.7

Associations with past 12-month physical intimate partner violence victimization

In unadjusted logistic regression analyses for both sexes, older age, experience of hunger, substance use (tobacco and cannabis use), violence related behaviour (in a physical fight, carried a weapon, belonging to a violent group, and sexual violence victimization), sexual risk behaviour (early sexual debut, multiple sexual partners, and non-condom use at last sex), and high or multiple psychological distress were positively associated with past 12-month physical IPV victimization. Parental provision of necessities, non-truant school attendance and parental support were protective from past 12-month physical IPV victimization. In addition, among boys, being a religious or spiritual person was protective from past 12-month physical IPV victimization, and among girls, being bullied was positively associated with past 12-month physical IPV victimization (see Table 2).

Table 2. Unadjusted logistic regression analysis with physical IPV victimization

	All	Male	Female
Variable	UOR (95% CI)	UOR (95% CI)	UOR (95% CI)
Sociodemographics			
Age in years			
≤11-14	1 (Reference)	1 (Reference)	1 (Reference)
15-16	1.14 (0.86, 1.52)	0.86 (0.56, 1.33)	1.72 (1.15, 2.56)**
17-18 or more	1.40 (1.04, 1.90)*	1.19 (0.72, 1.97)	1.84 (1.13, 2.98)*
Sex			
Female	1 (Reference)	---	---
Male	1.28 (0.97, 1.65)		
Parents provide necessities	0.48 (0.34, 0.68)***	0.44 (0.29, 067)***	0.53 (0.35, 0.82)**
Experience hunger	1.83 (1.07, 3.13)*	1.51 (0.78, 2.93)	2.11 (0.93, 4.76)
Risk behaviour			
Current tobacco use	2.10 (1.57, 2.81)***	2.22 (1.41, 3.49)***	1.81 (1.25, 2.62)**
Heavy alcohol use	1.23 (0.87, 1.73)	0.98 (0.64, 1.50)	1.59 (1.00, 2.52)
Current cannabis use	2.07 (1.25, 3.42)**	2.46 (1.34, 4.54)**	1.53 (0.67, 3.54)
In physical fight	1.48 (1.10, 1.99)**	1.35 (0.90, 2.01)	1.59 (0.99, 2.56)
Physically attacked	1.35 (0.95, 1.90)	1.20 (0.68, 2.13)	1.51 (0.92, 2.50)
Was bullied	1.35 (0.92, 1.97)	0.89 (0.55, 1.42)	2.04 (1.30, 3.22)**
Carried a weapon	2.10 (1.37, 3.20)***	1.83 (1.10, 3.04)*	2.43 (1.26, 4.69)**
Belongs to violent group	2.88 (1.98, 4.18)***	3.39 (1.95, 5.87)***	2.05 (0.87, 4.80)
Physical violence from parents	0.99 (0.60, 1.61)	1.22 (0.67, 2.25)	0.82 (0.41, 1.65)
Sexual violence victimization	1.77 (1.17, 2.68)**	2.32 (1.02, 5.28)*	1.71 (1.06, 2.75)*
Early sexual debut (<14 years)	2.29 (1.62. 3.25)***	2.15 (1.31, 3.53)**	2.36 (1.23, 4.53)**
Multiple sexual partners	2.09 (1.56, 2.81)***	1.98 (1.29, 3.04)**	2.17 (1.53, 3.08)***
Non-condom use at last sex	2.12 (1.47, 3.05)***	1.86 (1.04, 3.34)*	2.47 (1.61, 3.79)***

Table 2. (Continued)

	All	Male	Female
Variable	UOR (95% CI)	UOR (95% CI)	UOR (95% CI)
Psychological distress			
0	1 (Reference)	1 (Reference)	1 (Reference)
1	1.14 (0.83, 1.57)	1.29 (0.85, 1.96)	1.02 (0.62, 1.67)
2-5	1.60 (1.06, 2.44)*	1.05 (0.51, 2.14)	2.23 (1.31, 3.79)**
Protective factors			
School attendance	0.59 (0.45, 0.76)***	0.60 (0.42, 0.88)**	0.56 (0.40, 0.77)***
Religious person	0.79 (0.56, 1.12)	0.64 (0.41, 0.99)*	1.00 (0.67, 1.52)
Peer support	0.77 (0.55, 1.06)	0.85 (0.55, 1.30)	0.71 (0.44, 1.14)
Lives with both parents	0.98 (0.73, 1.32)	0.89 (0.60, 1.31)	1.03 (0.64, 1.66)
Parental support			
Low	1 (Reference)	1 (Reference)	1 (Reference)
Medium	0.55 (0.39, 0.77)***	0.73 (0.45, 1.16)	0.39 (0.23, 0.69)***
High	0.61 (0.44, 0.86)**	0.66 (0.42, 1.05)	0.59 (0.36, 0.94)*

UOR=Unadjusted odds ratio; ***P<0.001; **P<0.01; *P<0.05.

Table 3. Adjusted logistic regression analysis with physical IPV victimization

	All	Male	Female
Variable	AOR (95% CI)	AOR (95% CI)	AOR (95% CI)
Sociodemographics			
Age in years			
≤11-14	1 (Reference)	---	1 (Reference)
15-16	1.11 (0.78, 1.56)		1.32 (0.82, 2.11)
17-18 or more	1.19 (0.82, 1.73)		1.19 (0.68, 2.09)
Parents provide necessities	0.58 (0.38, 0.87)**	0.57 (0.34, 0.96)*	0.65 (0.37, 1.12)
Experience hunger	1.00 (0.46, 2.14)	---	---
Risk behaviour			
Current tobacco use	1.16 (0.73, 1.83)	0.93 (0.46, 1.86)	---
Current cannabis use	1.09 (0.56, 2.10)	(1.28 (0.48, 3.39)	---
In physical fight	1.09 (0.74, 1.59)	---	---
Was bullied	---	---	1.82 (1.07, 3.10)*
Carried a weapon	---	1.12 (0.58, 2.16)	1.75 (0.99, 3.11)
Belongs to violent group	1.83 (0.97, 3.45)	2.72 (1.19, 6.19)*	---
Physical violence from parents			
Sexual violence victimization	0.98 (0.53, 1.81)	1.16 (0.20, 6.82)	0.91 (0.51, 1.64)
Early sexual debut (<14 years)	1.66 (1.00, 2.77)*	1.56 (0.77, 3.19)	1.47 (0.68, 3.19)
Multiple sexual partners	1.21 (0.78, 1.86)	1.43 (0.84, 2.43)	1.21 (0.68, 2.12)
Non-condom use at last sex	1.44 (0.97, 2.15)	1.24 (0.61, 2.51)	1.80 (1.07, 3.03)*

	All	Male	Female
Variable	AOR (95% CI)	AOR (95% CI)	AOR (95% CI)
Psychological distress			
0	1 (Reference)	---	1 (Reference)
1	1.11 (0.75, 1.62)		0.79 (0.46, 1.34)
2-5	1.26 (0.78, 2.02)		1.31 (0.78, 2.23)
Protective factors			
School attendance	0.79 (0.56, 1.11)	0.77 (0.45, 1.32)	0.70 (0.45, 1.09)
Religious person	---	0.75 (0.47, 1.20)	---
Parental support			
Low	1 (Reference)	---	1 (Reference)
Medium	0.73 (0.48, 1.12)		0.45 (0.24, 0.86)*
High	1.04 (0.69, 1.57)		0.98 (0.52, 1.85)

AOR=Adjusted odds ratio; ***P<0.001; **P<0.01; *P<0.05.

In adjusted logistic regression analyses between both sexes, parental provision of necessities was negatively and early sexual debut was positively associated with past 12-month physical IPV victimization. In addition, among boys, belonging to a violent group was associated with recent physical IPV victimization, while among girls, being bullied and non-condom use at last sex were positively and medium parental support was negatively associated with recent physical IPV victimization (see Table 3).

DISCUSSION

The study found a prevalence of 10.5% (11.6% among boys and 9.4% among girls) past 12-month physical IPV victimization among school-going adolescents in Curaçao. These figures seem to compare with prevalence estimates among adolescents in the USA (7.8% - 13.5%) (2-5), and are lower than those found in South Africa (12.4% - 39.0%) (7, 8). Among boys, belonging to a violent group and inadequate parental provision of necessities and among girls, carried a weapon, non-condom use at last sex and lack of parental support were associated recent physical IPV victimization. These results seem to suggest potentially different risk factors at force between sexes. Further qualitative research is indicated to investigate how specific gender-role stereotypes in Curaçao cultures promote or discourage violence among intimate partners.

Previous studies found an association between older age and physical IPV victimization among adolescents (4, 10), while in this study this was only found in unadjusted analysis. This study found a similar prevalence of physical IPV victimization among boys and girls, which was also found among studies in American adolescents (4-6), while other studies found mixed results (7, 11). Among adults in Curaçao, IPV victimization was significantly higher among females than among males (9). More research is needed to explore the finding of non-significant sex differences in physical IPV victimization among adolescents in Curaçao.

This study found a protective effect of parental provision of necessities, in particular among boys, from physical IPV victimization. It may be important to consider this result in prevention programmes against physical IPV victimization. Several studies (10, 12) found an association between alcohol use and physical IPV victimization among adolescents, but this study did not find any association in Curaçao. In the unadjusted analyses, current tobacco and cannabis use were associated with physical IPV victimization, while a previous study did find an association between illicit drug use and physical IPV victimization (10).

This study also found that violence related behaviour (among boys, belonging to a violent group, and among girls bullying victimization) was associated with physical IPV victimization. These results are in agreement with previous studies (5, 12, 13). No associations between other violence related behaviours (physical fighting, sexual violence victimization, being a victim of violence by an adult in the household) and physical IPV victimization were found in this study, unlike in some previous studies (2-4).

As found in previous studies (3, 15, 16), this study found that early sexual debut and among girls that non-condom use at last sex increased the likelihood for physical IPV victimization. In addition, in unadjusted analysis, having multiple sexual partners was associated with physical IPV victimization, as also found in previous investigations (3, 10).

In previous studies (3-5), psychological distress was positively associated with physical IPV victimization among adolescents, while in this study this was only the case for girls in the unadjusted analyses. While some previous studies (2, 12) found that support from friends and parents and religious service attendance was protective from physical IPV victimization, this study only found medium parental support among girls protective, but in unadjusted analysis parental support and school attendance was protective, and among boys, being a religious or spiritual person was protective from physical IPV victimization. Parental monitoring has been found to protect from physical IPV victimization, perhaps because of a decreased likelihood of being in unsupervised social situations (2). In a recent review (12), several promising interventions to prevent physical IPV victimization among adolescents have been suggested, including "school-based dating violence interventions, community-based interventions to form gender equitable attitudes among boys and girls and parenting interventions and interventions with children and adolescents subjected to maltreatment."

Study limitations

The GSHS is limited to participants attending school, which excludes out-off school adolescents. The questionnaire was administered by self-report, and therefore some of the responses may have been biased; especially sexual risk behaviours and physical IPV victimization may have been underreported. The survey data were cross-sectional; therefore, no causal conclusions can be drawn. The study only covered physical IPV victimization. To gain a more comprehensive view into IPV, future studies should assess different types (physical, sexual and emotional) and frequency of both IPV victimization and perpetration.

Conclusion

More than one in ten school-going adolescents had been victim of physical IPV. Both boys and girls had experienced physical IPV victimization, but seemed to have a different risk profile, among boys, belonging to a violent group and inadequate parental provision of necessities and among girls, carried a weapon, non-condom use at last sex and lack of parental support were associated with physical IPV victimization. Interventions to prevent physical IPV victimization in this population may include multiple levels, including school-, community- and parent-based interventions.

Appendix 1. Description of Variables Used in This Study

Variables	Question	Response options (Coding scheme)
	Outcome variable	
Physical partner violence victimization	"During the past 12 months, did your boyfriend or girlfriend ever hit, slap, or physically hurt you on purpose?"	"Yes, No"
	Sociodemographic factors	
Age	"How old are you?"	"11 years old or younger to 18 years old or older"
Sex	"What is your sex?"	"Male, Female"
Provision of necessities	"During the past 30 days, how often did your parents or guardians provide for your necessities?"	"1= never to 5= always (coded 1–3=0 and 4–5=1)"
Hunger	"During the past 30 days, how often did you go hungry because there was not enough food in your home?"	"1= never to 5= always (coded 1–3=0 and 4–5=1)"
	Risk behaviour	
Current tobacco use	"During the past 30 days, on how many days did you smoke cigarettes/use any tobacco products other than cigarettes, such as cigars, cigarillos, or electronic cigarettes?"	"1=0 days to 7=All 30 days (coded 1=0 and 2-7=1)"
Heavy alcohol use (2 or more/day)	"During the past 30 days, on the days you drink alcohol, how many drinks did you usually drink per day?"	"1 = Not drink in the past 30 days to 7 = 5 or more drinks (coded 1–3 = 0 and 4–7 = 1)"

Variables	Question	Response options (Coding scheme)
	Risk behaviour	
Current cannabis use	"During the past 30 days, how many times have you used marijuana (also called weed, pot, cannabis, ganja, or grass)?"	"1=0 days to 7=All 30 days (coded 1=0 and 2-7=1)"
In a physical fight	"During the past 12 months, how many times were you in a physical fight?"	"1=0 times to 8=12 or more times (coded 1=0 and 2–8=1)"
Physically attacked	"During the past 12 months, how many times were you physically attacked?"	"1=0 times to 8=12 or more times (coded 1=0 and 2–8=1)"
Was bullied	"During the past 30 days, on how many days were you bullied?"	"1=0 days to 7=all 30 days (coded 1=0 and 2-7=1)"
Carried a weapon	"During the past 30 days, on how many days did you carry a weapon, such as a gun, knife, club, or brass knuckles?"	"1=0 days to 5=6 or more days) (coded 1=0 and 2-6=1)"
Belong to violent group	"Do you belong to any violent group?"	"Yes, No"
Physical violence from parents	"During the past 12 months, did your parents or guardians ever hit, slap, or physically hurt you on purpose?"	"Yes, No (coded yes=1 and no=0)"
Sexual violence victimization	"Have you ever been forced to have sexual intercourse when you did not want to?"	"Yes, No" (coded yes=1 and no=0)
Early sexual debut (<14 years)	"How old were you when you had sexual intercourse for the first time?"	"I have never had sexual intercourse, 11 years old or younger to 18 years old or older" (coded 11-13 years=1 and 14-18 years and never=0)"
Multiple sexual partners	"During your life, with how many people have you had sexual intercourse?"	"I have never had sexual intercourse, 1 person to 6 or more people" (coded 2-6 people=1 and never and 1=0)"
Non-condom use at last sex	"The last time you had sexual intercourse, did you or your partner use a condom or a rubber?"	"I have never had sexual intercourse, Yes, No (coded yes=0 and no=1)"
	Psychological distress	
No close friends	"How many close friends do you have?"	"1 = 0 to 4 = 3 or more (coded 1+=0, 0=1)"
Anxiety	"During the past 12 months, how often have you been so worried about something that you could not sleep at night?"	"1=never to 5=always (coded 1–3=0 and 4–5=1)"
Loneliness	"During the past 12 months, how often have you felt lonely?"	"1=never to 5=always (coded 1–3=0 and 4–5=1)"

Appendix 1. (Continued)

Variables	Question	Response options (Coding scheme)
	Psychological distress	
Suicide ideation	"During the past 12 months, did you ever seriously consider attempting suicide?"	"Yes, No"
Suicide attempt	"During the past 12 months, how many times did you actually attempt suicide?"	"1=0 times to 5=6 or more times (coded 1=0 and 2–5=1)"
	Protective factors	
School attendance	"During the past 30 days, on how many days did you miss classes or school without permission?"	"1=0 days to 5= 10 or more days (coded 1=0 and 2–5=1)"
Religious or spiritual person	"Do you think of yourself as a religious or spiritual person?"	"Yes, No"
Peer support	"During the past 30 days, how often were most of the students in your school kind and helpful?"	"1=never to 5=always (coded 1–3=0 and 4–5=1)"
Lives with both parents	"Which adult family members do you live with?"	1=both my mother and father to 5=I do not live with any adult family members (coded 2-5=0 and 1=1)
Parental supervision	"During the past 30 days, how often did your parents or guardians check to see if your homework was done?"	"1=never to 5=always (coded 1–3=0 and 4–5=1)"
Parental connectedness	"During the past 30 days, how often did your parents or guardians understand your problems and worries?"	"1=never to 5=always (coded 1–3=0 and 4–5=1)"
Parental bonding	"During the past 30 days, how often did your parents or guardians really know what you were doing with your free time?	"1=never to 5=always (coded 1–3=0 and 4–5=1)"
Parental respect for privacy	"During the past 30 days, how often did your parents or guardians go through your things without your approval?"	"1=never to 5=always (coded 1–3=0 and 4–5=1)"

REFERENCES

[1] World Health Organization. Preventing intimate partner and sexual violence against women: Taking action and generating evidence. Geneva: WHO, 2010.

[2] Howard D, Qiu Y, Boekeloo B. Personal and social contextual correlates of adolescent dating violence. J Adolesc Health 2003;33(1):9-17.

[3] Howard DE, Wang MQ, Yan F. Psychosocial factors associated with reports of physical dating violence victimization among US adolescent males. Adolescence 2008;43(171):449-60.

[4] Ramisetty-Mikler S, Goebert D, Nishimura S, Caetano R. Dating violence victimization: associated drinking and sexual risk behaviors of Asian, Native Hawaiian, and Caucasian high school students in Hawaii. J Sch Health 2006;76(8):423-9.

[5] Yan FA, Howard DE, Beck KH, Shattuck T, Hallmark-Kerr M. Psychosocial correlates of physical dating violence victimization among Latino early adolescents. J Interpers Violence 2010;25(5):808-31. doi: 10.1177/0886260509336958.

[6] Rothman EF, Xuan Z. Trends in physical dating violence victimization among U.S. high school students, 1999-2011. J Sch Violence 2014;13(3):277-90.

[7] Mason-Jones AJ, De Koker P, Eggers SM, Mathews C, Temmerman M, Leye E, De Vries PJ, De Vries H. Intimate partner violence in early adolescence: The role of gender, socioeconomic factors and the school. S Afr Med J 2016;106(5):60. doi: 10.7196/SAMJ.2016.v106i5.9770.

[8] Russell M, Cupp PK, Jewkes RK, Gevers A, Mathews C, LeFleur-Bellerose C, et al. Intimate partner violence among adolescents in Cape Town, South Africa. Prev Sci 2014;15(3):283-95. doi: 10.1007/s11121-013-0405-7.

[9] van Wijk NP, de Bruijn JG. Risk factors for domestic violence in Curaçao. J Interpers Violence 2012;27(15):3032-53.

[10] Rivera-Rivera L, Allen-Leigh B, Rodríguez-Ortega G, Chávez-Ayala R, Lazcano-Ponce E. Prevalence and correlates of adolescent dating violence: baseline study of a cohort of 7,960 male and female Mexican public school students. Prev Med 2007;44(6):477-84.

[11] Vagi KJ, O'Malley Olsen E, Basile KC, Vivolo-Kantor AM. Teen dating violence (physical and sexual) among US high school students: Findings from the 2013 National Youth Risk Behavior Survey. JAMA Pediatr 2015;169(5):474-82. doi: 10.1001/jamapediatrics.2014.3577.

[12] Lundgren R, Amin A. Addressing intimate partner violence and sexual violence among adolescents: emerging evidence of effectiveness. J Adolesc Health 2015;56(1 Suppl):S42-50. doi: 10.1016/j.jadohealth.2014.08.012.

[13] Gover AR, Jennings WG, Tewksbury R Adolescent male and female gang members' experiences with violent victimization, dating violence, and sexual assault. Am J Crim Justice 2009;34:103–15.

[14] Earnest AA, Brady SS. Dating violence victimization among high school students in minnesota: associations with family violence, unsafe schools, and resources for support. J Interpers Violence 2016;31(3):383-406. doi: 10.1177/0886260514555863.

[15] Eaton DK, Davis KS, Barrios L, Brener ND, Noonan RK. Associations of dating violence victimization with lifetime participation, co-occurrence, and early initiation of risk behaviors among U.S. high school students. J Interpers Violence 2007;22(5):585-602.

[16] Gonzalez-Guarda RM, Williams JR, Merisier M, Cummings AM, Prado G. Acculturation, risk behaviors and physical dating violence victimization among Cuban-American adolescents. J Pediatr Nurs 2014;29(6):633-40. doi: 10.1016/j.pedn.2014.03.001.

[17] World Health Organization (WHO) Global School-based Student Health Survey. Curaçao 2015 fact sheet. URL: https://www.who.int/ncds/surveillance/gshs/2015_Curaçao_GSHS_Fact_Sheet.pdf.

[18] Verstraeten S. National report the Curaçao Global School-based Student Health Survey (GSHS) study 2015. URL: https://www.who.int/ncds/surveillance/gshs/Final_report_2015_GSHS_Curaçao.pdf.

[19] World Health Organization (WHO). Global School-based Student Health Survey (GSHS). 2015 Curaçao GSHS Questionnaire. URL: https://www.who.int/ncds/surveillance/gshs/2015_GSHS_Curaçao_Questionnaire.pdf.

In: Adolescence in Curaçao
Editors: Soraya Verstraeten et al.
ISBN: 978-1-53617-522-6

Chapter 7

EFFECTS OF RECENT PHYSICAL PARTNER VIOLENCE VICTIMIZATION ON HEALTH RISK BEHAVIOURS AND MENTAL HEALTH AMONG A NATIONAL SAMPLE OF IN-SCHOOL ADOLESCENTS IN CURAÇAO

Karl Peltzer[1], PhD and Supa Pengpid[1,2,*], DrPH
[1]Department of Research Administration and Development, University of Limpopo, Turfloop, South Africa
[2]ASEAN Institute for Health Development, Mahidol University, Salaya, Phutthamonthon, Nakhon Pathom, Thailand

ABSTRACT

In this chapter we investigate the effects of physical intimate partner violence (IPV) victimization among adolescents in Curaçao. In the cross-

* ***Correspondence***: Professor Supa Pengpid, ASEAN Institute for Health Development, Mahidol University, 25/25 Phutthamonthon Road 4, Salaya, Phutthamonton, Nakhon Pathom 73170, Thailand. Email: supaprom@yahoo.com.

sectional Curaçao "Global School-Based Student Health Survey (GSHS)" in 2015, 2,765 adolescents (median age 15 years) responded to questions on sociodemographic factors, risk behaviours, violence, mental health, substance use and protective factors. The prevalence of past 12-month physical IPV victimization was 10.5%, 11.6% among boys and 9.4% among girls. In adjusted logistic regression analyses among both sexes, physical IPV victimization was associated with sexual risk behaviour (ever sex, early sexual debut, having had multiple sexual partners, non-condom use at last sex and adolescent pregnancy), violence related behaviour (carried a weapon and belonged to a violent group), poor mental health (sucide plan and suicide attempt) and current tobacco use. In addition, among boys, physical IPV victimization was associated with transactional sex, and among girls physical IPV victimization was associated with having been bullied. Recent physical IPV victimization was associated with sexual risk behaviours, including pregnancy, violence related behaviours, poor mental health and substance use. Interventions programmes targeting victimized adolescents should address linked health risk behaviours identified.

INTRODUCTION

Intimate partner violence (IPV) and other violence among adolescents is being increasingly recognized as common and having a wide range of health, behavioural and well-being consequences (1). Various studies have identified that a history physical IPV victimization among male and/or female adolescents is associated with sexual risk behaviours, violence related behaviours, poor mental health and substance use. Sexual risk behaviour among adolescents may include, currently sexually active (2), ever sex (3), early sexual debut (4, 5), multiple sexual partners (2, 4-6), no condom use at last sex (5, 6), and pregnancy (5, 6). Violence-related behaviours among adolescents may include in a physical fight (2), carried a weapon (2) and bullied (2).

Poor mental health as a consequence of physical IPV victimization among adolescents may include depression (7, 8), posttraumatic stress (7), suicide ideation (2, 5, 8, 9), suicide plan (2) and suicide attempt (2, 5). Several studies found that a history of physical IPV victimization among adolescents increased the odds for substance use, such as alcohol use (3), binge drinking (2), heavy smoking (5), current cannabis use (2), drug use (3), ever used cocaine (2, 5), and substance use at last sex (4). In order to better understand the context of the negative effects of physical IPV victimization among adolescents in a Caribbean setting, the study aimed to assess the effects of physical IPV victimization among adolescents in Curaçao.

OUR STUDY

Cross-sectional data from the 2015 Curaçao GSHS were analyzed (10). The study used a two-stage cluster sampling design to generate a representative sample of all students enrolled in public secondary education, comparable to US Grades 1-6, in Curaçao. "At the first stage, 28 schools were selected with probability proportional to enrolment size, and at the second stage, 161 classes were randomly selected" (11). All students in selected classes were eligible to participate after ethical approval *in accordance with the "WMA Declaration of Helsinki – Ethical Principles for Medical Research Involving Human Subjects"* and other permissions were granted and written informed consent was obtained from parents and children; the overall response rate was 83% (11).

Measures

The GSHS questionnaire applied to this analysis was used in this survey (see Appendix 1) (12). Past 12-month physical partner violence victimization was assessed with the question: "During the past 12 months, did your boyfriend or girlfriend ever hit, slap, or physically hurt you on purpose?" (Yes, No). Parental support (4 items) was categorized into 0-1 low, 2 medium and 3-4 high support. Psychological distress was defined as zero, single as one and multiple as 2-5 psychological distress, including the items loneliness, having no close friends, anxiety, suicidal ideation and suicide attempt.

Data analysis

Data analysis was conducted with "STATA software version 15.0 (Stata Corporation, College Station, TX, USA)", considering the complex study design. Multivariable logistic regression was used to assess the associations between physical IPV victimization, relevant confounders (age, sex, hunger, and parental provision of necessities, living status, school attendance, peer and parental support) and dependent variables (18 health risk behaviours and five poor mental health indicators). Missing data were excluded from the analysis. P values <0.05 were considered significant.

FINDINGS

The sample consisted of 2,765 school-going adolescents, 51.1% female and 48.9% male, 3.8% had mostly or always experienced hunger in the past month, 81.7% had parents or guardians that provided them mostly or always with necessities, 47.6% had peer support, 48.9% lived with both parents and 46.1% had high parental support. Overall, the prevalence of past 12-month physical IPV victimization was 10.5%, 11.6% among boys and 9.4% among girls.

Associations between physical IPV victimization and health risk behaviour

In adjusted logistic regression analyses among both sexes, physical IPV victimization was associated with sexual risk behaviour (ever sex, early sexual debut, having had multiple sexual partners, non-condom use at last sex and adolescent pregnancy), violence related behaviour (carried a weapon and belonged to a violent group), poor mental health (sucide plan and suicide attempt) and current tobacco use. In addition, among boys, physical IPV victimization was associated with transactional sex, and among girls physical IPV victimization was associated with having been bullied (see Table 1).

Table 1. Effects of physical IPV victimization on risk behaviours and mental health

Variable	All	Male	Female
	AOR (95% CI)[1]	AOR (95% CI)[1]	AOR (95% CI)[1]
Sexual risk behaviour			
Ever sex	1.52 (1.12, 2.07)**	1.17 (0.76, 1.81)	2.05 (1.43, 2.93)***
Early sexual debut (<14 years)	2.03 (1.29, 3.21)**	2.12 (1.19, 3.79)*	1.92 (0.98, 3.77)
Forced sexual intercourse	1.16 (0.73, 1.83)	0.65 (0.12, 3.39)	1.27 (0.77, 2.08)
Multiple sexual partners	1.86 (1.40, 2.48***	1.77 (1.11, 2.83)*	1.94 (1.35, 2.79)***
Transactional sex	2.15 (0.87, 5.31)	3.15 (1.13, 8.75)*	1.07 (0.25, 4.60)
Non-condom use at last sex	1.83 (1.28, 2.63)***	1.38 (0.68, 2.81)	2.38 (1.55, 3.67)***
Non-birth control use at last sex	1.18 (0.82, 1.71)	1.08 (0.68, 1.72)	1.20 (0.72, 2.00)
Adolescent pregnancy	1.92 (1.03, 3.60)*	2.22 (0.71, 6.97)	1.81 (0.88, 3.73)
Violence related behaviour			
In physical fight	1.34 (0.91, 1.96)	1.14 (0.64, 2.05)	1.60 (0.90, 2.63)
Physically attacked	1.01 (0.66, 1.53)	0.71 (0.33, 1.54)	1.25 (0.71, 2.19)
Carried a weapon	1.82 (1.14, 2.88)*	1.48 (0.83, 2.64)	2.30 (1.28, 4.12)**
Belong to violent group	2.48 (1.52, 4.03)***	3.35 (1.60, 6.99)**	1.78 (0.69, 4.61)
Was bullied	1.32 (0.87, 1.99)	0.79 (0.47, 1.34)	2.02 (1.22, 3.34)**
Physical violence from parents	0.80 (0.49, 1.31)	1.04 (0.50, 2.17)	0.65 (0.34, 1.22)
Mental health			
Anxiety	1.18 (0.79, 1.76)	0.48 (0.16, 1.42)	1.60 (0.93, 2.74)
Loneliness	1.00 (0.66, 1.52)	0.81 (0.41, 1.59)	1.21 (0.73, 2.00)
Suicide ideation	1.38 (0.98, 1.89)	1.24 (0.59, 2.59)	1.49 (0.97, 2.28)
Suicide plan	1.97 (1.32, 2.94)***	2.51 (1.24, 5.08)*	1.70 (1.01. 2.84)*
Suicide attempt	1.61 (1.04, 2.48)*	2.38 (1.16, 4.86)*	1.30 (0.72, 2.96)
Substance use			
Heavy alcohol use	1.09 (0.77, 1.64)	0.80 (0.44, 1.45)	1.39 (0.79, 2.44)
Current tobacco use	1.91 (1.35, 2.70)***	1.86 (1.00, 3.47)	1.81 (1.22. 2.69)**
Current cannabis use	1.69 (0.98, 2.92)	1.94 (0.85, 4.45)	1.38 (0.56, 3.44)
Used methamphetamine, cocaine, or XTC one or more times	2.41 (0.90, 6.45)	1.77 (0.36, 8.78)	2.78 (0.87, 8.89)

AOR = Adjusted Odds Ratio; ***P < 0.001; **P < 0.01; *P < 0.05;

[1]Adjusted for age, hunger, parental provision of necessities, living status (with both parents), school attendance, peer and parental support.

Discussion

Consistent with findings of various previous studies (2-8), this study found among both boys and girls that had experienced recent physical IPV victimization had an increased likelihood of five of eight sexual risk behaviours, including pregnancy, two of six violence related behaviours, two of five poor mental health indicators and one of four substance use types. These findings replicate earlier results showing the wide range of possible effects of physical IPV victimization on various health risk behaviours and poor mental indicators among adolescents (5, 6), which makes them vulnerable to HIV infection, other sexually transmitted infection, and unwanted pregnancy.

Further, the study also found gender specific effects of physical IPV victimization, e.g., among boys transactional sex and belonging to a violent group and among girls bullying victimization and tobacco use. It is possible that boys who have experienced physical IPV engage more likely in transactional sex and join a violent group, and victimized girls become also target of bullying and try to cope by using tobacco. Unlike some previous studies (2, 3, 5), this study did not find an association between physical IPV victimization and heavy alcohol use, cannabis and other drug use. The study also failed to find an association between physical IPV victimization and in a physical fight and suicide ideation, as found in several previous studies (2, 5, 8, 9). Programmes targeting the prevention of physical IPV victimization among adolescents should include multiple risk behaviours, including sexual risk behaviour, violence related activities and substance use.

Study Limitations

The GSHS is limited to participants attending school, which does not include out-off school adolescents. The questionnaire administered was by self-report, and therefore some of the responses may have been biased;

especially sexual risk behaviours and physical IPV victimization among both males and females, may have been underreported. The survey data were limited to cross-sectional. For example, it remains unclear what mechanism or chronology was involved in relation to physical IPV victimization and pregnancy, e.g., if physical IPV victimization led to the inability to use condoms, if the abusive partner actively prevented contraception use or if the abused feared using condoms. The study only assessed physical IPV victimization, and future studies should assess different types (physical, sexual and emotional) and severity of IPV victimization.

CONCLUSION

More than one in ten school-going adolescents had been victim of physical IPV. Both boys and girls had experienced physical IPV victimization, but seemed to have a different risk profile, among boys, belonging to a violent group and inadequate parental provision of necessities and among girls, carried a weapon, non-condom use at last sex and lack of parental support were associated with physical IPV victimization. Interventions to prevent physical IPV victimization in this population may include multiple levels, including school-based, community-based and parenting interventions.

REFERENCES

[1] Stark L, Seff I, Hoover A, Gordon R, Ligiero D, Massetti G. Sex and age effects in past-year experiences of violence amongst adolescents in five countries. PLoS One 2019;14(7):e0219073. doi: 10.1371/journal.pone.0219073. eCollection 2019.

[2] Vagi KJ, O'Malley Olsen E, Basile KC, Vivolo-Kantor AM. Teen dating violence (physical and sexual) among US high school students: Findings from the 2013 National Youth Risk Behavior Survey. JAMA Pediatr 2015;169(5):474-82. doi: 10.1001/jamapediatrics.2014.3577.

[3] Lormand DK, Markham CM, Peskin MF, Byrd TL, Addy RC, Baumler E, Tortolero SR. Dating violence among urban, minority, middle school youth and associated

sexual risk behaviors and substance use. J Sch Health 2013;83(6):415-21. doi: 10.1111/josh.12045.

[4] Alleyne B, C oleman-Cowger VH, Crown L, Gibbons MA, Vines LN. The effects of dating violence, substance use and risky sexual behavior among a diverse sample of Illinois youth. J Adolesc 2011;34(1):11-8. doi: 10.1016/j.adolescence.2010.03.006.

[5] Silverman JG, Raj A, Mucci LA, Hathaway JE. Dating violence against adolescent girls and associated substance use, unhealthy weight control, sexual risk behavior, pregnancy, and suicidality. JAMA 2001;286(5):572-9.

[6] Silverman JG, Raj A, Clements K. Dating violence and associated sexual risk and pregnancy among adolescent girls in the United States. Pediatrics 2004;114(2): e220-5.

[7] Holmes K, Sher L. Dating violence and suicidal behavior in adolescents. Int J Adolesc Med Health 2013;25(3):257-61. doi: 10.1515/ijamh-2013-0059.

[8] Banyard VL, Cross C. Consequences of teen dating violence: understanding intervening variables in ecological context. Violence Against Women 2008;14(9):998-1013. doi: 10.1177/1077801208322058.

[9] Nahapetyan L, Orpinas P, Song X, Holland K. Longitudinal association of suicidal ideation and physical dating violence among high school students. J Youth Adolesc 2014;43(4):629-40. doi: 10.1007/s10964-013-0006-6.

[10] World Health Organization (WHO) Global School-based Student Health Survey (GSHS). 2015 Curacao. URL: https://www.who.int/ncds/surveillance/gshs/curacaodataset/en/.

[11] Verstraeten S. National report the Curaçao Global School-based Student Health Survey (GSHS) study 2015. URL: https://www.who.int/ncds/surveillance/gshs/Final_report_2015_GSHS_Curacao.pdf.

[12] World Health Organization (WHO) Global School-based Student Health Survey (GSHS). 2015 Curacao GSHS Questionnaire. URL: https://www.who.int/ncds/surveillance/gshs/2015_GSHS_Curacao_Questionnaire.pdf.

APPENDIX 1. DESCRIPTION OF VARIABLES USED IN THIS STUDY

Variables	Question	Response options (Coding scheme)
Physical partner violence victimization	"During the past 12 months, did your boyfriend or girlfriend ever hit, slap, or physically hurt you on purpose?"	"Yes, No (coded yes = 1 and no = 0)"
	Sociodemographic and protective factors	
Age	"How old are you?"	"11 years old or younger to 18 years old or older"
Sex	"What is your sex?"	"Male, Female"
Hunger	"During the past 30 days, how often did you go hungry because there was not enough food in your home?"	"1 = never to 5 = always (coded 1–3 = 0 and 4–5 = 1)"
Provision of necessities	"During the past 30 days, how often did your parents or guardians provide for your necessities?"	"1 = never to 5 = always (coded 1–3 = 0 and 4–5 = 1)"
Lives with both parents	"Which adult family members do you live with?"	"1 = both my mother and father to 5 = I do not live with any adult family members (coded 2-5 = 0 and 1 = 1)"
School attendance	"During the past 30 days, on how many days did you miss classes or school without permission?"	"1 = 0 days to 5 = 10 or more days (coded 1 = 0 and 2–5 = 1)"
Peer support	"During the past 30 days, how often were most of the students in your school kind and helpful?"	"1 = never to 5 = always (coded 1–3 = 0 and 4–5 = 1)"
Parental supervision	"During the past 30 days, how often did your parents or guardians check to see if your homework was done?"	"1 = never to 5 = always (coded 1–3 = 0 and 4–5 = 1)"
Parental connectedness	"During the past 30 days, how often did your parents or guardians understand your problems and worries?"	"1 = never to 5 = always (coded 1–3 = 0 and 4–5 = 1)"
Parental bonding	"During the past 30 days, how often did your parents or guardians really know what you were doing with your free time?	"1 = never to 5 = always (coded 1–3 = 0 and 4–5 = 1)"
Parental respect for privacy	"During the past 30 days, how often did your parents or guardians go through your things without your approval?"	"1 = never to 5 = always (coded 1–3 = 0 and 4–5 = 1)"

Appendix 1. (Continued)

Variables	Question	Response options (Coding scheme)
	Sexual risk behaviour	
Ever sex	"Have you ever had sexual intercourse?"	"Yes, No (coded yes = 1 and no = 0)"
Early sexual debut (<14 years)	"How old were you when you had sexual intercourse for the first time?"	"I have never had sexual intercourse, 11 years old or younger to 18 years old or older" (coded 11-13 years = 1 and 14-18 years and never = 0)"
Forced sexual intercourse	"Have you ever been forced to have sexual intercourse when you did not want to?"	"Yes, No" (coded yes = 1 and no = 0)
Multiple sexual partners	"During your life, with how many people have you had sexual intercourse?"	"I have never had sexual intercourse, 1 person to 6 or more people" (coded 2-6 people = 1 and never and 1 = 0)"
Transactional sex	"During your life, have you ever had sexual intercourse in exchange for something, such as a phone, jewelry, or money?"	"I have never had sexual intercourse, Yes, No (coded yes = 1 and no = 0)"
Non-condom use at last sex	"The last time you had sexual intercourse, did you or your partner use a condom or a rubber?"	"I have never had sexual intercourse, Yes, No (coded yes = 0 and no = 1)"
Non-birth control at last sex	"The last time you had sexual intercourse, did you or your partner use any other method of birth control, such as withdrawal, rhythm (safe time), birth control pills, or any other method to prevent pregnancy?"	"I have never had sexual intercourse, Yes, No (coded yes = 0 and no = 1)"
Adolescent pregnancy	"How many times have you been pregnant or gotten someone pregnant?"	"1 = 0 times to 3 = 2 or more times Coded (coded 1 = 0 and 2-3 = 1)"
	Violence related behaviour	
In a physical fight	"During the past 12 months, how many times were you in a physical fight?"	"1 = 0 times to 8 = 12 or more times (coded 1 = 0 and 2–8 = 1)"

Variables	Question	Response options (Coding scheme)
	Violence related behaviour	
Physically attacked	“During the past 12 months, how many times were you physically attacked?”	“1 = 0 times to 8 = 12 or more times (coded 1 = 0 and 2–8 = 1)”
Carried a weapon	“During the past 30 days, on how many days did you carry a weapon, such as a gun, knife, club, or brass knuckles?”	“1 = 0 days to 5 = 6 or more days) (coded 1 = 0 and 2-6 = 1)”
Belong to violent group	”Do you belong to any violent group?”	“Yes, No (coded yes = 1 and no = 0)”
Was bullied	“During the past 30 days, on how many days were you bullied?”	“1 = 0 days to 7 = all 30 days (coded 1 = 0 and 2-7 = 1)”
Physical violence from parents	“During the past 12 months, did your parents or guardians ever hit, slap, or physically hurt you on purpose?”	“Yes, No (coded yes = 1 and no = 0)”
	Mental health	
Anxiety	“During the past 12 months, how often have you been so worried about something that you could not sleep at night?”	“1 = never to 5 = always (coded 1–3 = 0 and 4–5 = 1)”
Loneliness	“During the past 12 months, how often have you felt lonely?”	“1 = never to 5 = always (coded 1–3 = 0 and 4–5 = 1)”
Suicide ideation	“During the past 12 months, did you ever seriously consider attempting suicide?”	“Yes, No”
Suicide plan	“During the past 12 months, did you make a plan about how you would attempt suicide?”	“Yes, No”
Suicide attempt	“During the past 12 months, how many times did you actually attempt suicide?”	“1 = 0 times to 5 = 6 or more times (coded 1 = 0 and 2–5 = 1)”
	Substance use	
Heavy alcohol use (2 or more/day)	“During the past 30 days, on the days you drink alcohol, how many drinks did you usually drink per day?”	“1 = Not drink in the past 30 days to 7 = 5 or more drinks (coded 1–3 = 0 and 4–7 = 1)”
Current tobacco use	“During the past 30 days, on how many days did you smoke cigarettes/use any tobacco products other than cigarettes, such as cigars, cigarillos, or electronic cigarettes?”	“1 = 0 days to 7 = All 30 days (coded 1 = 0 and 2-7 = 1)”

Appendix 1. (Continued)

Variables	Question	Response options (Coding scheme)
	Substance use	
Current cannabis use	"During the past 30 days, how many times have you used marijuana (also called weed, pot, cannabis, ganja, or grass)?"	"1 = 0 days to 7 = All 30 days (coded 1 = 0 and 2-7 = 1)"
Lifetime methamphetamine, etc. use	"During your life, how many times have you used methamphetamine, cocaine, or XTC (also called speed, base, rock, crack, and uppers)?"	1 = 0 times to 5 = 20 or more times (coded 1 = 0 and 2-5 = 1)

In: Adolescence in Curaçao
Editors: Soraya Verstraeten et al.
ISBN: 978-1-53617-522-6

Chapter 8

PREVALENCE AND ASSOCIATED FACTORS OF WEAPON CARRYING AMONG IN-SCHOOL ADOLESCENTS IN CURAÇAO: A CROSS-SECTIONAL NATIONAL SURVEY

Karl Peltzer[1], PhD and Supa Pengpid[1,2,*], DrPH
[1]Department of Research Administration and Development, University of Limpopo, Turfloop, South Africa
[2]ASEAN Institute for Health Development, Mahidol University, Salaya, Phutthamonthon, Nakhon Pathom, Thailand

ABSTRACT

In this chapter we aimed to assess the prevalence and correlates of recent weapon carring among a nationally representative sample of school adolescents in Curaçao. In the cross-sectional Curaçao "Global School-Based Student Health Survey (GSHS)" in 2015, 2,765 adolescents

* ***Correspondence***: Professor Supa Pengpid, ASEAN Institute for Health Development, Mahidol University, 25/25 Phutthamonthon Road 4, Salaya, Phutthamonton, Nakhon Pathom 73170, Thailand. E-Mail: supaprom@yahoo.com.

(median age 15 years) responded to questions on sociodemographic factors, various risk behaviours, psychological distress, and protective factors. The prevalence of past-month weapon carrying was 13.9%, 18.1% among boys and 9.5% among girls. In adjusted logistic regression analysis among both sexes, male sex, current tobacco use, heavy alcohol use, in a physical fight, belonging to a violent group, having had multiple sexual partners, having sustained a serious injury, and multiple psychological distress was associated with past-month weapon carrying. In addition, among boys, having been physically attacked was positively and school attendance was negatively associated with past-month weapon carrying, and among girls, current cannabis use was positively and living with both parents and high parental support were negatively associated with past-month weapon carrying. Almost one in five boys and one in ten girls had been carrying a weapon. Results identified a potentionally high-risk group of adolescents (males, substance use, violence, sexual risk behaviour, and injury) that could be targeted for strategies to reduce weapon carrying in this population.

INTRODUCTION

Youth violence is a global public health problem, and weapon carrying by adolescents is an important risk behaviour for violence among youth (1). In an investigation among school-going adolescents in the United States Virgin Islands, 15% had carried a weapon in the past month (2), in the US based national "Youth Risk Behavior Survey," 6.5% reported past 30 days weapon carrying onto school property (3), and the past 12 month prevalence of weapon carrying among school students in Bangkok, Thailand, was 7.8% (4). In five countries of the "Health Behaviour in School Aged Children Survey," the prevalence of past month weapon carrying was the highest in the US (22.2% among boys and 7.1% among girls) and the lowest in French Belgium (11.3% among boys and 1.6% among girls) (5). There is a lack of data on weapon carrying among adolescents and its correlates in the Caribbean, such as in Curaçao.

Risk factors for weapon carrying among adolescents (male and/or females) may include sociodemographic factors, substance use, violence-related behaviour, sexual risk behaviour, psychological distress and protective factors. Sociodemographic factors include males (2, 4), middle or older age (4, 6), and ethnicity (3). Substance related risk factors include tobacco use (2, 3, 4), alcohol use (3, 4), and illicit drug use (2, 4). Violence related factors for weapon carrying among adolescents include violence perpetration and victimization (6, 7), engaged in physical fighting (3, 4), having threatened or injuried (3), history of forced sexual intercourse (3), partner violence (6), witnessing violence (6), and associating with delinquent peers (7). Stayton et al. (8) found relationship between sexual risk behaviour, such as having multiple sexual partners, and weapon carrying among adolescents.

Several studies found a link between psychological distress, such as suicidal ideation (3), suicide attempt, suicide plan (4), depression (3), and weapon carrying among adolescents. Moreover, some studies also identified protective factors from weapon carrying among adolescents, including interpersonal connectedness (6), school connectedness (6), and greater parental warmth (7). The study aimed to assess the prevalence and associated factors of recent weapon carring among a nationally representative sample of in-school adolescents in Curaçao.

OUR STUDY

Cross-sectional data from the 2015 Curaçao GSHS were analyzed (9). The study utilized a two-stage cluster sampling design to generate representative data of all students enrolled in public secondary education, comparable to US Grades 1-6, in Curaçao. "At the first stage, 28 schools were selected with probability proportional to enrolment size, and at the second stage, 161 classes were randomly selected" (10). All students in selected classes were eligible to participate after ethical approval *in accordance with the "WMA Declaration of Helsinki – Ethical Principles for Medical Research Involving Human Subjects"* and other permissions were granted and written informed consent was obtained from parents and children; the overall response rate was 83% (10).

Measures

The GSHS questionnaire applied to this analysis was used in this survey (see appendix 1) (11). Past month weapon carrying was assessed with the question: "During the past 30 days, on how many days did you carry a weapon, such as a gun, knife, club, or brass knuckles?" (Number of days). Parental support (four items) was categorized into 0-1 low, 2 medium and 3-4 high support. Psychological distress was defined as zero, single as one and multiple as 2-5 psychological distress, including the items loneliness, having no close friends, anxiety, suicidal ideation and suicide attempt.

Data analysis

Data analysis was conducted with "STATA software version 15.0 (Stata Corporation, College Station, TX, USA)", considering the complex study design. Frequency tabulations were used to describe the sample. Logistic regression was used to assess the associations between independent variables (sociodemographic factors, substance use, violence-related behaviour, sexual risk behaviour, psychological distress, and protective factors) and past-month weapon carrying. Variables which found significant at $P < 0.05$ in bivariate analysis were included in the multivariable model, overall, and for boys and girls separately. Missing data were excluded from the analysis. P values <0.05 were considered significant.

FINDINGS

The sample consisted of 2,765 school-going adolescents, 51.1% female and 48.9% male, 3.8% had experienced food insecurity or hunger in the past month, and 81.7% had parents or guardians that provided them mostly or always with necessities. More than two thirds (69.0%) of students

Table 1. Sample and weapon carrying characteristics

Variable	Sample	Weapon carrying in the past 30 days		
	Total	All	Male	Female
	N (%)	%	%	%
All	2765	13.9	18.1	9.5
Sociodemographics				
Age in years				
≤11-14	1054 (32.8)	12.9	15.4	9.1
15-16	824 (32.7)	15.6	22.1	9.5
17-18 or more	877 (34.5)	13.3	18.1	8.9
Parents provide necessities	2082 (81.7)	12.4	16.7	8.4
Experience hunger	102 (3.8)	27.0	28.8	16.2
Risk behaviour				
Current tobacco use	345 (13.2)	38.3	44.7	27.4
Heavy alcohol use	477 (19.0)	26.3	35.6	16.4
Current cannabis use	136 (5.7)	39.7	44.3	32.1
In physical fight	492 (17.9)	28.8	31.4	23.9
Physically attacked	394 (14.3)	21.0	26.0	15.4
Was bullied	683 (25.4)	20.2	23.4	15.8
Physical intimate partner violence victimization	282 (10.5)	22.6	26.9	17.3
Belongs to violent group	165 (6.1)	37.8	40.1	32.6
Physical violence from parents	417 (15.2)	22.1	32.8	13.0
Forced sexual intercourse	159 (5.9)	14.9	26.7	14.3
Early sexual debut (<14 years)	230 (9.3)	27.8	26.7	25.9
Multiple sexual partners	480 (19.5)	24.3	30.0	16.1
Injured	808 (31.7)	22.2	24.9	17.2
Psychological distress				
0	1715 (65.1)	10.1	13.9	5.4
1	531 (20.5)	16.8	26.5	8.5
2-5	379 (14.4)	21.7	26.2	19.6
Protective factors				
School attendance	1976 (73.4)	10.9	14.0	8.0
Religious person	1717 (69.0)	12.4	15.8	9.3
Peer support	1241 (47.6)	11.3	15.4	7.7
Lives with both parents	1325 (48.9)	11.5	15.6	7.0
Parental support				
Low	665 (27.2)	18.8	21.0	16.0
Medium	659 (26.7)	13.6	18.6	8.8
High	1167 (46.1)	9.5	14.3	5.4

perceived themselves to be a religious or spiritual person, 73.4% attended school in the past month, 47.6% received mostly or always peer support in the past 30 days and 46.1% scored high on parental support. The prevalence of various risk behaviours, psychological distress and protective factors are described in table 1. Overall, the prevalence of past-month weapon carrying was 13.9%, 18.1% among boys and 9.5% among girls (see Table 1).

Associations with past-month weapon carrying

In unadjusted logistic regression analysis for both sexes, experience of hunger, substance use (tobacco use, heavy alcohol use and cannabis use), violence related behaviour (physically attacked, in a physical fight, was bullied, physical intimate partner violence victimization, belonging to a violent group, and physical violence from parents), sexual risk behaviour (early sexual debut and multiple sexual partners), injury and psychological distress were positively associated with past-month weapon carrying. Parental provision of necessities, school attendance, peer support, living with both parents and parental support were protective from past-month weapon carrying. Similar results were found when analysing boys and girls separately (see Table 2).

In adjusted logistic regression analysis among both sexes, male sex, current tobacco use, heavy alcohol use, in a physical fight, belonging to a violent group, having had multiple sexual partners, having sustained a serious injury, and multiple psychological distress was associated with past-month weapon carrying. In addition, among boys, having been physically attacked was positively and school attendance was negatively associated with past-month weapon carrying, and among girls, current cannabis use was positively and living with both parents and high parental support were negatively associated with past-month weapon carrying (see Table 3).

Table 2. Unadjusted associations with weapon carrying in the past 30 days

Variable	All	Male	Female
	UOR (95% CI)	UOR (95% CI)	UOR (95% CI)
Sociodemographics			
Age in years			
≤11-14	1 (Reference)	1 (Reference)	1 (Reference)
15-16	1.25 (0.92, 1.70)	1.56 (1.05, 2.31)*	1.05 (0.62, 1.76)
17-18 or more	1.04 (0.73, 1.47)	1.21 (0.81, 1.80)	0.97 (0.61, 1.55)
Parents provide necessities	0.64 (0.45, 0.91)*	0.75 (0.51, 1.11)	0.60 (0.38, 0.96)*
Experience hunger	2.38 (1.52, 3.74)***	1.85 (0.95, 3.61)	1.98 (1.02, 3.86)*
Risk behaviour			
Current tobacco use	5.56 (4.12, 7.13)***	5.17 (3.75, 7.13)***	5.28 (3.13, 8.91)***
Heavy alcohol use	2.83 (2.20, 3.63)***	3.28 (2.35, 4.57)***	2.39 (1.50, 3.81)***
Current cannabis use	5.00 (3.40, 7.36)***	4.22 (2.42, 7.37)***	5.71 (3.11, 10.51)***
In physical fight	3.41 (2.56, 4.54)***	2.69 (1.87, 3.86)***	4.20 (2.89, 6.10)***
Physically attacked	1.83 (1.39, 2.41)***	1.71 (1.18, 2.28)**	2.05 (1.31, 3.22)**
Was bullied	1.95 (1.54, 2.45)***	1.56 (1.15, 2.12)**	2.60 (1.85, 3.65)***
Physical intimate partner violence victimization	2.10 (1.37, 3.20)***	1.83 (1.10, 3.04)*	2.43 (1.26, 4.69)**
Belongs to violent group	4.46 (2.95, 6.78)***	3.46 (2.04, 5.85)***	5.63 (3.28, 9.65)***
Physical violence from parents	2.18 (1.61, 2.93)***	2.72 (1.82, 4.13)***	1.74 (1.08, 2.92)*
Forced sexual intercourse	1.55 (0.83, 2.91)	1.78 (0.79, 3.61)	1.76 (0.83, 3.72)
Early sexual debut (<14 years)	2.86 (2.20, 3.71)***	1.88 (1.26, 2.81)**	4.10 (2.42, 6.29)***
Multiple sexual partners	2.64 (1.93, 3.60)***	2.60 (1.79, 3.78)***	2.23 (1.40, 3.66)***
Injured	2.85 (2.38, 3.39)***	2.12 (1.54, 2.72)***	3.42 (2.38, 4.90)***

Table 2. (Continued)

Variable	All	Male	Female
	UOR (95% CI)	UOR (95% CI)	UOR (95% CI)
Psychological distress			
0	1 (Reference)	1 (Reference)	1 (Reference)
1	1.80 (1.33, 2.43)***	2.24 (1.52, 3.29)***	1.65 (0.95, 2.87)
2-5	2.47 (1.67, 3.68)***	2.19 (1.19, 4.02)*	4.32 (2.66, 7.02)***
Protective factors			
School attendance	0.48 (0.38, 0.61)***	0.43 (0.33, 0.56)***	0.62 (0.40,)*
Religious person	0.83 (0.64, 1.08)	0.72 (0.52, 1.01)	1.11 (0.71, 1.72)
Peer support	0.72 (0.58, 0.89)**	0.75 (0.55, 1.03)	0.72 (0.43, 1.20)
Lives with both parents	0.68 (0.53, 0.88)**	0.66 (0.46, 0.94)*	0.63 (0.43, 0.920*
Parental support			
Low	1 (Reference)	1 (Reference)	1 (Reference)
Medium	0.68 (0.49, 0.93)**	0.86 (0.55, 1.33)	0.51 (0.30, 0.84)**
High	0.46 (0.34, 0.61)***	0.63 (0.43, 0.91)*	0.30 (0.21, 0.44)***

UOR = Unadjusted odds ratio; ***P < 0.001; **P < 0.01; *P < 0.05.

Table 3. Adjusted associations with weapon carrying in the past 30 days

Variable	All	Male	Female
	AOR (95% CI)	AOR (95% CI)	AOR (95% CI)
Sociodemographics			
Sex			
Female	1 (Reference)	---	---
Male	1.96 (1.33, 2.88)***		
Age in years			
≤11-14	1 (Reference)	1 (Reference)	1 (Reference)
15-16	0.91 (0.55, 1.50)	0.98 (0.53, 1.79)	0.94 (0.44, 1.99)
17-18 or more	0.95 (0.51, 1.76)	0.89 (0.44, 1.82)	1.12 (0.50, 2.49)
Parents provide necessities	1.24 (0.71, 2.16)	1.12 (0.58, 2.18)	1.33 (0.68, 2.59)
Experience hunger	0.60 (0.28, 1.28)	0.84 (0.32, 2.22)	0.27 (0.06, 1.29)
Risk behaviour			
Current tobacco use	2.12 (1.38, 3.27)***	2.60 (1.39, 4.88)***	1.47 (0.82, 2.65)
Heavy alcohol use	1.81 (1.21, 2.70)**	2.45 (1.38, 4.38)**	1.30 (0.69, 2.43)
Current cannabis use	1.42 (0.63, 3.19)	0.92 (0.31, 2.78)	2.56 (1.01, 6.53)*
In physical fight	1.78 (1.20, 2.64)**	1.64 (0.96, 2.80)	2.13 (1.14, 3.98)*
Physically attacked	1.23 (0.74, 2.06)	1.86 (1.02, 3.40)*	0.87 (0.38, 2.01)
Was bullied	1.25 (0.87, 1.80)	1.20 (0.77, 1.87)	1.33 (0.78, 2.27)
Physical intimate partner violence victimization	1.26 (0.73, 2.20)	1.00 (0.48, 2.09)	1.62 (0.85, 3.12)
Belongs to violent group	2.96 (1.39, 6.32)**	2.38 (0.84, 6.77)	4.02 (1.67, 9.68)**
Physical violence from parents	1.10 (0.72, 1.69)	1.53 (0.78, 2.98)	0.63 (0.32, 1.22)
Early sexual debut (<14 years)	1.27 (0.77, 2.09)	0.84 (0.43, 1.63)	1.73 (0.83, 3.60)
Multiple sexual partners	1.65 (1.04, 2.62)*	2.21 (1.09, 4.50)*	1.19 (0.60, 2.37)
Injured	1.86 (1.36, 2.53)***	1.47 (0.92, 2.34)	2.65 (1.69, 4.17)***

Table 3. (Continued)

Psychological distress			
0	1 (Reference)	1 (Reference)	1 (Reference)
1	1.50 (0.95, 2.39)	2.05 (1.23, 3.41)**	1.00 (0.42, 2.38)
2-5	1.52 (1.01, 2.28)*	1.13 (0.50, 2.58)	1.69 (0.90, 3.18)
Protective factors			
School attendance	0.67 (0.44, 1.02)	0.51 (0.32, 0.82)**	0.92 (0.47, 1.80)
Peer support	0.77 (0.55, 1.02)	0.84 (0.54, 1.30)	0.61 (0.34, 1.09)
Lives with both parents	0.84 (0.61, 1.15)	0.94 (0.59, 1.50)	0.58 (0.36, 0.94)*
Parental support			
Low	1 (Reference)	1 (Reference)	1 (Reference)
Medium	1.13 (0.69, 1.84)	1.08 (0.55, 2.10)	1.11 (0.59, 2.09)
High	0.97 (0.64, 1.46)	1.50 (0.81, 2.77)	0.50 (0.28, 0.87)*

AOR = Unadjusted odds ratio; ***P < 0.001; **P < 0.01; *P < 0.05.

Discussion

The study found a prevalence of 13.9% (18.1% among boys and 9.5% among girls) past-month weapon carrying among school-going adolescents in Curaçao. These figures are similar to a study among school adolescents in the United States Virgin Islands (15%) (2), and in a recent study in the US (22.2% among boys and 7.1% among girls) (5), but higher than in an older study in the US (6.5%) (3), and Thailand (7.8% past 12 months) (4).

Consistent with previous studies (2, 4), this study found that male sex was associated with weapon carrying. This sex difference may be attributed to various reasons, including the perception that other students are carrying weapons, and being more likely to engage in substance use and violence-related behaviour than females (3). Unlike some previous studies (4, 6), this study did not find significant age differences in the prevalence weapon carrying.

This study found that current tobacco use and heavy alcohol use, and among girls current cannabis use, were associated with weapon carrying. These findings concur with several previous studies (2-4). In agreement with previous studies (3, 4, 7), this study found that violence-related behaviour (in a physical fight and belonging to a violent group) and having been injured were associated with weapon carrying. In a separate analysis (not shown), it was found that among students who had sustained a serious injury from a gunshot wound, 52.4% had been carrying a weapon. This result underlines the importance of carrying a weapon and possible injury. Unlike some previous studies (3, 6), this study did not find an association between a history of forced sexual intercourse, partner violence (6), and weapon carrying. However, this study seems to confirm an association between sexual risk behaviour, such as having multiple sexual partners, and weapon carrying among adolescents (8).

In agreement with several studies (3, 4), this study found an association between psychological distress, including suicidal behaviour, and weapon carrying among adolescents. This result may indicate a clustering of risk behaviours with substance use, and violence-related behaviours (3). Therefore, interventions may need to target multiple risk behaviours. Moreover, some studies found gender specific differences (6, 8), which was in this study among boys school connectedness and among girls living with both parents and high parental support. Interventions may utilize these gender specific protective factors from weapon carrying.

Study Limitations

The GSHS is limited to participants attending school, which does not include out-off school adolescents. The questionnaire administered was by self-report, and therefore some of the responses may have been biased; especially carrying a weapon among both males and females, may have been underreported. The survey data were cross-sectional so that no causal conclusions can be drawn. The study only assessed carrying a weapon with one question, and more details about different contexts could be assessed in future studies.

Conclusion

Almost one in five boys and one in ten girls had been carrying a weapon. Results identified a potentionally high-risk group of adolescents (males, substance use, violence, sexual risk behaviour, and injury) that could be targeted for strategies to reduce weapon carrying in this population. In addition, sex specific protective factors (school attendance for boys and living with both parents and high parental support for girls) were identified for weapon carrying, which should be utilized in gender specific interventions.

APPENDIX 1. DESCRIPTION OF VARIABLES USED IN THIS STUDY

Variables	Question	Response options (Coding scheme)
	Sociodemographic factors	
Age	"How old are you?"	"11 years old or younger to 18 years old or older"
Sex	"What is your sex?"	"Male, Female"
Provision of necessities	"During the past 30 days, how often did your parents or guardians provide for your necessities?"	"1 = never to 5 = always (coded 1–3 = 0 and 4–5 = 1)"
Hunger	"During the past 30 days, how often did you go hungry because there was not enough food in your home?"	"1 = never to 5 = always (coded 1–3 = 0 and 4–5 = 1)"
	Outcome variable	
Weapon carrying	"During the past 30 days, on how many days did you carry a weapon, such as a gun, knife, club, or brass knuckles?"	"1 = 0 days to 5 = 6 or more days"
	Risk behaviour	
Current tobacco use	"During the past 30 days, on how many days did you smoke cigarettes/use any tobacco products other than cigarettes, such as cigars, cigarillos, or electronic cigarettes?"	"1 = 0 days to 7 = All 30 days (coded 1 = 0 and 2-7 = 1)"
Heavy alcohol use (2 or more/day)	"During the past 30 days, on the days you drink alcohol, how many drinks did you usually drink per day?"	"1 = Not drink in the past 30 days to 7 = 5 or more drinks (coded 1–3 = 0 and 4–7 = 1)"
Current cannabis use	"During the past 30 days, how many times have you used marijuana (also called weed, pot, cannabis, ganja, or grass)?"	"1 = 0 days to 7 = All 30 days (coded 1 = 0 and 2-7 = 1)"
In a physical fight	"During the past 12 months, how many times were you in a physical fight?"	"1 = 0 times to 8 = 12 or more times (coded 1 = 0 and 2–8 = 1)"
Physically attacked	"During the past 12 months, how many times were you physically attacked?"	"1 = 0 times to 8 = 12 or more times (coded 1 = 0 and 2–8 = 1)"
Was bullied	"During the past 30 days, on how many days were you bullied?"	"1 = 0 days to 7 = all 30 days (coded 1 = 0 and 2-7 = 1)"

Appendix 1. (Continued)

Variables	Question	Response options (Coding scheme)
Partner violence	"During the past 12 months, did your boyfriend or girlfriend ever hit, slap, or physically hurt you on purpose?"	"Yes, No"
Belong to violent group	"Do you belong to any violent group?"	"Yes, No"
Physical violence from parents	"During the past 12 months, did your parents or guardians ever hit, slap, or physically hurt you on purpose?"	"Yes, No (coded yes = 1 and no = 0)"
Forced sexual intercourse	"Have you ever been forced to have sexual intercourse when you did not want to?"	"Yes, No" (coded yes = 1 and no = 0)"
Early sexual debut (<14 years)	"How old were you when you had sexual intercourse for the first time?"	"1 = never to 8 = 18 years old or older"
Multiple sexual partners	"During your life, with how many people have you had sexual intercourse?"	"I have never had sexual intercourse, 1 person to 6 or more people" (coded 2-6 people = 1 and never and 1 = 0)"
Injury	"During the past 12 months, how many times were you seriously injured?"	1 = 0 times to 8 = 12 or more times (coded 1 = 0 and 2–8 = 1)
	Psychological distress	
No close friends	"How many close friends do you have?"	"1 = 0 to 4 = 3 or more (coded 1+ = 0, 0 = 1)"
Anxiety	"During the past 12 months, how often have you been so worried about something that you could not sleep at night?"	"1 = never to 5 = always (coded 1–3 = 0 and 4–5 = 1)"
Loneliness	"During the past 12 months, how often have you felt lonely?"	"1 = never to 5 = always (coded 1–3 = 0 and 4–5 = 1)"
Suicide ideation	"During the past 12 months, did you ever seriously consider attempting suicide?"	"Yes, No"

Variables	Question	Response options (Coding scheme)
Suicide attempt	"During the past 12 months, how many times did you actually attempt suicide?"	"1 = 0 times to 5 = 6 or more times (coded 1 = 0 and 2–5 = 1)"
	Protective factors	
School attendance	"During the past 30 days, on how many days did you miss classes or school without permission?"	"1 = 0 days to 5 = 10 or more days (coded 1 = 1 and 2–5 = 0)"
Religious or spiritual person	"Do you think of yourself as a religious or spiritual person?"	"Yes, No"
Peer support	"During the past 30 days, how often were most of the students in your school kind and helpful?"	"1 = never to 5 = always (coded 1–3 = 0 and 4–5 = 1)"
Lives with both parents	"Which adult family members do you live with?"	1 = both my mother and father to 5 = I do not live with any adult family members (coded 2-5 = 0 and 1 = 1)
Parental supervision	"During the past 30 days, how often did your parents or guardians check to see if your homework was done?"	"1 = never to 5 = always (coded 1–3 = 0 and 4–5 = 1)"
Parental connectedness	"During the past 30 days, how often did your parents or guardians understand your problems and worries?"	"1 = never to 5 = always (coded 1–3 = 0 and 4–5 = 1)"
Parental bonding	"During the past 30 days, how often did your parents or guardians really know what you were doing with your free time?	"1 = never to 5 = always (coded 1–3 = 0 and 4–5 = 1)"
Parental respect for privacy	"During the past 30 days, how often did your parents or guardians go through your things without your approval?"	"1 = never to 5 = always (coded 1–3 = 0 and 4–5 = 1)"

REFERENCES

[1] Krug EG, Mercy JA, Dahlberg LL, Zwi AB. The world report on violence and health. Lancet 2002;360(9339):1083-8.

[2] Lloyd JJ, Delva J, Arria AM. Recent weapon carrying and substance use among United States Virgin Islands youth. Subst Use Misuse 2000;35(9):1207-25.

[3] Muula AS, Rudatsikira E, Siziya S. Correlates of weapon carrying among high school students in the United States. Ann Gen Psychiatry 2008;7:8. doi: 10.1186/1744-859X-7-8.

[4] Saiphoklang OA, Wongboonsin K, Wongboonsin P, Perngparn U, Cottler LB. The association between weapon carrying and health risk behaviors among adolescent students in Bangkok, Thailand. J Interpers Violence 2017;32(20):3111-3130. doi: 10.1177/0886260515596977.

[5] Walsh SD, Molcho M, Craig W, Harel-Fisch Y, Huynh Q, Kukaswadia A, et al. Physical and emotional health problems experienced by youth engaged in physical fighting and weapon carrying. PLoS One 2013;8(2):e56403. doi: 10.1371/journal.pone.0056403.

[6] Kodjo CM, Auinger P, Ryan SA. Demographic, intrinsic, and extrinsic factors associated with weapon carrying at school. Arch Pediatr Adolesc Med 2003;157(1):96-103.

[7] Stickley A, Koyanagi A, Koposov R, Blatný M, Hrdlička M, Schwab-Stone M, et al. Correlates of weapon carrying in school among adolescents in three countries. Am J Health Behav 2015;39(1):99-108. doi: 10.5993/AJHB.39.1.11.

[8] Stayton C, McVeigh KH, Olson EC, Perkins K, Kerker BD. Victimization and health risk factors among weapon-carrying youth. Am J Health Behav 2011;35(6):654-63.

[9] World Health Organization (WHO) Global School-based Student Health Survey (GSHS). 2015 Curacao. URL: https://www.who.int/ncds/surveillance/gshs/curacaodataset/en/.

[10] Verstraeten S. National report the Curaçao Global School-based Student Health Survey (GSHS) study 2015. URL: https://www.who.int/ncds/surveillance/gshs/Final_report_2015_GSHS_Curacao.pdf.

[11] World Health Organization (WHO) Global School-based Student Health Survey (GSHS). 2015 Curacao GSHS Questionnaire. URL: https://www.who.int/ncds/surveillance/gshs/2015_GSHS_Curacao_Questionnaire.pdf.

In: Adolescence in Curaçao
Editors: Soraya Verstraeten et al.
ISBN: 978-1-53617-522-6

Chapter 9

HIGH ALCOHOL USE AND MISUSE AMONG BOTH BOYS AND GIRLS IN A NATIONAL SAMPLE OF SCHOOL ADOLESCENTS IN CURAÇAO

Karl Peltzer*[1], *PhD and Supa Pengpid*[1,2,*], *DrPH
[1]Department of Research Administration and Development, University of Limpopo, Turfloop, South Africa
[2]ASEAN Institute for Health Development, Mahidol University, Salaya, Phutthamonthon, Nakhon Pathom, Thailand

ABSTRACT

In this chapter we aim to investigate the prevalence and correlates of alcohol use and misuse among adolescents in the 2016 Curaçao "Global School-Based Student Health Survey (GSHS)." In all, 2,765 adolescents with a median age of 15 years (interquartile range=3) from Curaçao

[*] ***Correspondence***: Professor Supa Pengpid, ASEAN Institute for Health Development, Mahidol University, 25/25 Phutthamonthon Road 4, Salaya, Phutthamonton, Nakhon Pathom 73170, Thailand. E-Mail: supaprom@yahoo.com.

responded to the 2015 cross-sectional GSHS. Results indicate that 40.8% of the adolescents (43.8% among females and 38.0% among males) reported past-month alcohol use, 21.6% ever been drunk, and 19.0% past-month heavy alcohol use (≥two more drinks/day). In adjusted logistic regression analysis, older age, female sex, parental tobacco use, exposure to secondary smoke, current tobacco use, ever cannabis use, multiple sexual partners, school truancy, soft drink consumption, injury, psychological distress, and lack of parental support were associated with alcohol use and/or misuse. A high prevalence of alcohol use and misuse was found and strategies to prevent alcohol misuse, including a number of risk behaviours, are needed.

INTRODUCTION

Particularly, adolescents are vulnerable to alcohol use, which may increase health risks in later life (1). Based on the "Global School-Based Student Health Survey (GSHS)" in 27 countries in the Americas, the prevalence of past-month alcohol use was 34.9%, and lifetime drunkenness 22.2% among young adolescents (12-15 years) (2). The prevalence of past-month alcohol use was 52.4%, and lifetime drunkenness 36.5% among young adolescents (12-15 years) in Jamaica, and 31.5% current alcohol use and 21.3% ever drunk in Trinidad and Tobago (2). In a recent survey among school adolescents in Ghana, the prevalence of current alcohol consumption was 12.6% and lifetime drunkenness 11.1% (3). In the 2017 Curaçao national adult health survey, 57.6% were alcohol users (4). National data on alcohol consumption pattern and its associated factors among adolescents are lacking for Curaçao.

Factors associated with alcohol use and misuse among adolescents, may include, as reviewed in Pengpid and Peltzer (5), male sex, older age, lower economic status, psychological distress, legal and illegal drug use, parental substance use, sexual risk behaviour, school truancy, interpersonal violence, injury and low or inadequate peer and parental support. This study aimed to assess the prevalence and correlates of alcohol use and misuse among school adolescents in Curaçao.

OUR STUDY

Cross-sectional data from the 2015 Curaçao GSHS were analysed (6). The study used a two-stage cluster sample design to produce data representative of all students enrolled in public secondary education, comparable to US Grades 1-6, in Curaçao. "At the first stage, 28 schools were selected with probability proportional to enrolment size, and at the second stage, 161 classes were randomly selected" (7). All students in selected classes were eligible to participate after ethical approval **in accordance** *with the "WMA Declaration of Helsinki – Ethical Principles for Medical Research Involving Human Subjects"* and other permissions were granted and informed consent was obtained from parents and children; the overall response rate was 83% (7).

Measures

The questionnaire items used in this paper are described in appendix 1. "The psychological distress items (no close friends, loneliness, anxiety, suicidal ideation and suicide attempt) were summed, and grouped into 0=0 low, 1=1 medium and 2-5=2 high. The four items on parental or guardian support (supervision, connectedness, bonding and respect for privacy) were summed, and classified into three groups, 0-1= low, 2= medium and 3-4= high support" (5).

Data analysis

Descriptive statistics was used to describe the sample and chi-square statistics to test differences in proportion. Adjusted logistic regression analyses were used to estimate the associations between independent variables and current alcohol use, ever been drunk and heavy alcohol use (≥two drinks/day) as dependent variables. Missing data were excluded from the analysis. $P < 0.05$ was considered significant. Considering the complex study design, all analyses were performed using STATA software version 15.0 (Stata Corporation, College Station, TX, USA).

FINDINGS

The sample included 2,765 school-going adolescents (median age 15 years, interquartile range 3 years), 51.1% were females and 48.9% males. The prevalence of current alcohol use was 40.8%, ever been drunk 21.6% and heavy drinking (≥2 drinks/day) in the past month 19.0%. Further sample details are shown in Table 1.

Table 1. Sample characteristics and alcohol use

Variable	Sample	Current alcohol use	Ever drunk	Two or more drinks/day
	N (%)	%	%	%
All	2765	40.8	21.6	19.0
Age (years)				
≤14	1054 (32.8)	22.7	10.2	7.6
15 or 16	828 (32.7)	43.8	20.6	19.5
≥17	877 (34.5)	54.4	33.3	29.3
Sex				
Female	1508 (51.1)	43.5	20.1	18.6
Male	1230 (48.9)	38.0	23.3	19.5
Hunger	102 (3.8)	38.8	26.4	18.9
Parental tobacco use	572 (21.2)	50.5	30.3	26.2
Secondary smoke	1599 (58.3)	51.6	27.6	25.6
Current tobacco use	345 (13.2)	78.4	53.0	46.9
Ever cannabis use	257 (10.9)	75.5	62.3	44.7
Sex partners (≥two)	480 (19.5)	68.5	48.0	40.5
Soft drink consumption	1670 (60.9)	47.0	22.8	22.3
School truancy	652 (26.6)	57.0	37.6	29.6
Bullied	683 (25.4)	47.4	24.6	22.7
In physical fight	492 (17.9)	51.9	30.4	24.9
Physically attacked	394 (14.3)	26.6	19.4	19.4
Injury	808 (31.7)	49.8	27.3	26.3
Psychological distress				
0	1719 (65.1)	37.1	18.8	17.6
1	531 (20.5)	42.2	21.8	18.1
2 or more	379 (14.4)	54.4	33.8	25.6

Variable	Sample	Current alcohol use	Ever drunk	Two or more drinks/day
	N (%)	%	%	%
Peer support	1241 (47.6)	40.5	20.5	20.3
Parental support				
0-1	665 (27.2)	49.8	30.7	26.0
2	659 (26.7)	42.6	23.0	20.1
3-4	1167 (46.1)	34.2	15.7	14.8

Table 2. Adjusted associations with alcohol use and misuse

Variable	Current alcohol use	Ever drunk	Two or more drinks/day
	AOR (95% CI)	AOR (95% CI)	AOR (95% CI)
Age (years)			
≤14	1 (Reference)	1 (Reference)	1 (Reference)
15 or 16	2.23 (1.75, 2.83)***	1.77 (1.25, 2.50)***	2.41 (1.63, 3.56)***
≥17	3.59 (2.61, 4.94)***	2.94 (2.00, 4.30)***	4.01 (2.63, 6.11)***
Sex			
Female	1 (Reference)	1 (Reference)	1 (Reference)
Male	0.59 (0.46, 0.76)***	1.12 (0.76, 1.63)	0.95 (0.69, 1.31)
Hunger	0.64 (0.33, 1.25)	0.65 (0.25, 1.67)	0.59 (0.23, 1.45)
Parental tobacco use	1.24 (0.91, 1.68)	1.45 (1.01, 2.08)*	1.33 (0.95, 1.87)
Secondary smoke	1.99 (1.56, 2.54)***	1.38 (0.99, 1.93)	1.94 (1.44, 2.61)***
Current tobacco use	4.78 (3.14, 7.26)***	2.22 (1.55, 3.18)***	2.72 (1.73, 4.28)***
Ever cannabis use	2.85 (1.79, 4.55)***	4.36 (3.01, 6.10)***	2.01 (1.26, 3.20)**
Sex partners (≥two)	1.97 (1.50, 2.58)***	2.15 (1.50, 3.08)***	1.77 (1.26, 2.50)***
Soft drink consumption	1.89 (1.49, 2.41)***	0.99 (0.74 1.32)	1.77 (1.37, 2.29)***
School truancy	1.46 (1.07, 1.99)*	1.60 (1.11, 2.31)*	1.46 (1.02, 2.10)*
Bullied	1.24 (0.95, 1.60)	1.17 (0.83, 1.63)	1.25 (0.91, 1.70)
In physical fight	1.62 (1.11, 2.36)*	1.62 (0.98, 2.66)	1.26 (0.87, 1.81)
Physically attacked	0.88 (0.60, 1.31)	1.13 (0.73, 1.77)	0.59 (0.36, 0.95)*
Injury	1.52 (1.17, 1.97)**	1.08 (0.82, 1.42)	1,75 (1.31, 2.35)***
Psychological distress			
0	1 (Reference)	1 (Reference)	1 (Reference)
1	0.93 (0.67, 1.29)	1.06 (0.81, 1.40)	0.85 (0.60, 1.19)
2 or more	1.04 (0.74, 1.47)	1.51 (1.04, 2.19)*	0.91 (0.52, 1.61)
Peer support	1.12 (0.90, 1.38)	0.94 (0.73, 1.22)	1.18 (0.89, 1.55)
Parental support			
0-1	1 (Reference)	1 (Reference)	1 (Reference)
2	0.86 (0.65, 1.14)	0.79 (0.57, 1.10)	0.79 (0.55, 1.15)
3-4	0.75 (0.55, 1.03)	0.67 (0.49, 0.93)*	0.65 (0.46, 0.91)*

AOR=Adjusted Odds Ratio; ***P<0.001; **P<0.01; *P<0.05.

In adjusted logistic regression analysis, older age was associated with alcohol use and misuse, female sex was associated with current alcohol use, and experiencing hunger was not significantly associated with alcohol use and misuse. Parental tobacco increased the odds for lifetime drunkenness, and secondary smoke exposure was associated with current alcohol use and heavy drinking. Current tobacco use, ever cannabis use as well as having had multiple sexual partners were highly significantly associated alcohol use and misuse. School truancy, in a physical fight and having sustained a serious injury was associated with at least one of the alcohol use indicators. Having multiple psychological distress increased the likelihood of lifetime drunkenness, and high parental support reduced the odds for lifetime drunkenness and heavy drinking (see Table 2).

DISCUSSION

The study found among in-school adolescents in the 2015 GSHS in Curaçao, a high prevalence of past-month alcohol use (40.8%) and alcohol misuse (lifetime drunkenness=21.6%, and heavy drinking=19.0%), which is higher than the pooled estimates from 27 countries in the Americas, in terms of past-month alcohol use (34.8%) but was similar regarding ever been drunk (22.2%) (2). The prevalence of current alcohol used and lifetime drunkenness was in this study lower than in Jamaica but higher than in Trinidad and Tobago (2), and Ghana (3), and almost similar to the adult current alcohol use rate in Curaçao (57.6%) (4).

Unlike previous studies (2, 8), this study found that the prevalence of alcohol use was significantly higher in females than in males. Consistent with previous studies (2, 9), in this study alcohol use and misuse significantly increased with age. Among those students who were past-month alcohol users, 30.3%, 23.7% and 13.8% obtained alcohol from their family, store and friends, respectively (analysis not shown), indicating that alcohol use among adolescents seem acceptable in Curaçao.

Consistent with previous studies (5, 9, 10), this survey found that a number of risk behaviours (current tobacco use, ever cannabis use, multiple sexual partners, school truancy, soft drink consumption, and injury) were correlated with current alcohol use and/or alcohol misuse. The clustering of various risk behaviours has been identified in previous studies (5, 10), in particular regarding different types of substance use but also truancy and sexual risk behaviour. The occurrence of several health risk behaviours identified in this study seems to confirm the "problem behaviour theory in vulnerable adolescents" (11). In agreement with previous studies (12, 13), this study found a correlation between psychological distress and ever drunk. Consistent with results from a previous study (9), this study found an association between parental tobacco use and drunkenness but not with current and heavy alcohol use. Consistent with some previous studies (5, 14), this study found that lack of parental support was correlated with ever drunk and heavy drinking. Intervention programmes may want to include an increase in parental or guardian supervision or monitoring of their adolescent children. There is a need for the development and implementation of a regional alcohol policy (15). In addition, school-based alcohol prevention interventions may be implemented, as they have been found effective in reducing alcohol misuse (16).

Study limitation

Study limitations include the cross-sectional nature of this investigation and the limitation of the sample to adolescents attending school. Peer and parental alcohol consumption were not measured in this study, and such measures should be part of future investigations.

CONCLUSION

The study found a high prevalence of past-month alcohol use, lifetime drunkenness and heavy alcohol use among both male and female school adolescents in Curaçao. Older age, female sex, parental tobacco use, exposure to secondary smoke, current tobacco use, ever cannabis use, multiple sexual partners, school truancy, soft drink consumption, injury, psychological distress, and lack of parental support were associated with alcohol use and/or misuse. Intervention efforts are indicated against alcohol use and misuse taking into account the clustered nature of various risk behaviours.

APPENDIX 1. VARIABLE DESCRIPTION

Variables	Question	Response options (coding scheme)
Age	"How old are you?"	11 years old or younger to 18 years old or older
Sex	"What is your sex?"	Male, Female
Hunger	"During the past 30 days, how often did you go hungry because there was not enough food in your home?"	1 = never to 5 = always (coded 1–3=0 and 4–5=1)
Alcohol use	"During the past 30 days, on how many days did you have at least one drink containing alcohol?"	1 = 0 days to 7 = All 30 days (coded 1=0 and 2-7=1)
	"During the past 30 days, on the days you drink alcohol, how many drinks did you usually drink per day?"	1=Not drink in the past 30 days to 7=5 or more drinks (coded 1-3=0 and 4-7=1)
	"During your life, how many times did you drink so much alcohol that you were really drunk?"	1=0 times and 4=10 or more times (coded 1=0 and 2-4=1)
Either or both parents use tobacco	"Which of your parents or guardians use any form of tobacco?"	1=neither, 2=my father or male guardian, 3=my mother or female guardian, 4=both
Secondary smoke	"During the past 7 days, on how many days have people smoked in your presence?"	1=0 days to 5=All seven days (coded 1=0 and 2-5=1)
Current tobacco use	During the past 30 days, on how many days did you smoke cigarettes/use any tobacco products other than cigarettes, such as cigars, cigarillos, or electronic cigarettes?"	1=0 days to 7=All 30 days (coded 1=0 and 2-7=1)
Cannabis use	"During your life, how many times have you used marijuana (also called weed, pot, cannabis, ganja, or grass)?"	1=0 times to 5=20 or more times (coded 1=0 and 2-5=1)
Sexual behaviour	"During your life, with how many people have you had sexual intercourse?"	1=I have never had to 7=6 or more people (coded 1-2=0 and 3-7=1)

Variables	Question	Response options (coding scheme)
Soft drink consumption	"During the past 30 days, how many times per day did you usually drink carbonated soft drinks, such as Coke, Sprite, fria, monster, busta, RedBull, coco rico, and malta? (Do not include diet soft drinks.)"	1=not in the past days to 7=5 or more times per day (coded 1-2=0 and 3-7=1)
School truancy	"During the past 30 days, on how many days did you miss classes or school without permission?"	1=0 days to 5= 10 or more days (coded 1=0 and 2–5=1)
Bullied	"During the past 30 days, on how many days were you bullied?"	1=0 days to 7=All 30 days (coded 1=0 and 2–7=1)
In a physical fight	"During the past 12 months, how many times were you in a physical fight?"	1=0 times to 8=12 or more times (coded 1=0 and 2–8=1)
Physically attacked	"During the past 12 months, how many times were you physically attacked?"	1=0 times to 8=12 or more times (coded 1=0 and 2–8=1)
Injury	"During the past 12 months, how many times were you seriously injured?"	1=0 times to 8=12 or more times (coded 1=0 and 2–8=1)
Psychological distress		
No close friends	"How many close friends do you have?"	1 = 0 to 4 = 3 or more (coded 1+=0, 0=1)
Anxiety	"During the past 12 months, how often have you been so worried about something that you could not sleep at night?"	1=never to 5=always (coded 1–3=0 and 4–5=1)
Loneliness	"During the past 12 months, how often have you felt lonely?"	1=never to 5=always (coded 1–3=0 and 4–5=1)
Suicide ideation	"During the past 12 months, did you ever seriously consider attempting suicide?"	Yes, No
Suicide attempt	"During the past 12 months, how many times did you actually attempt suicide?"	1=0 times to 5=6 or more times (coded 1=0 and 2–5=1)
Protective factors		
Peer support	"During the past 30 days, how often were most of the students in your school kind and helpful?"	1=never to 5=always (coded 1–3=0 and 4–5=1)
Parental connectedness	"During the past 30 days, how often did your parents or guardians understand your problems and worries?"	1=never to 5=always (coded 1–3=0 and 4–5=1)
Parental bonding	"During the past 30 days, how often did your parents or guardians really know what you were doing with your free time?	1=never to 5=always (coded 1–3=0 and 4–5=1)
Parental respect for privacy	"During the past 30 days, how often did your parents or guardians go through your things without your approval?"	1=never to 5=always (coded 1–3=0 and 4–5=1)

REFERENCES

[1] Nixon K, McClain JA. Adolescence as a critical window for developing an alcohol use disorder: current findings in neuroscience. Curr Opin Psychiatry 2010;23(3): 227-32.

[2] Ma C, Bovet P, Yang L, Zhao M, Liang Y, Xi B. Alcohol use among young adolescents in low-income and middle-income countries: A population-based study. Lancet Child Adolesc Health 2018;2(6):415-29.

[3] Asante KO, Kugbey N. Alcohol use by school-going adolescents in Ghana: Prevalence and correlates. Mental Health Prev 2019;13:75-81.

[4] Verstraeten SPA, Griffith M, Pin R. The National Health Survey Curaçao 2017. Results, methods and tables. Volksgezondheid Instituut Curaçao (VIC) Martinus Centrum Curaçao Molenplein z/n, Otrobanda, 2018. [Dutch].

[5] Pengpid S, Peltzer K. Alcohol use and misuse among school-going adolescents in Thailand: Results of a national survey in 2015. Int J Environ Res Public Health 2019;16(11): pii: E1898. doi: 10.3390/ijerph16111898.

[6] World Health Organization (WHO). Global School-based Student Health Survey (GSHS). URL: http://www.who.int/chp/gshs/en/.

[7] Verstraeten S. The Curaçao Global School-based Student Health Survey (GSHS). Willemstad: Volksgezondheid Instituut Curaçao, 2015.

[8] Abel WD, Weaver S, Ricketts Roomes T, Agu CF, Smith PW, Oshi DC, et al. Risk Factors Associated with Frequent Alcohol Binge Drinking among Jamaicans: Does Gender Matter? Asian Pac J Cancer Prev 2018;19(S1):39-44.

[9] Siziya S, Rudatsikira E, Muula AS. Alcohol use among school-going adolescents in Harare, Zimbabwe: results from the 2003 Global School-Based Health Survey. Tanzan J Health Res 2009;11(1):11-6.

[10] Faeh D, Viswanathan B, Chiolero A, Warren W, Bovet P. Clustering of smoking, alcohol drinking and cannabis use in adolescents in a rapidly developing country. BMC Public Health 2006;6:169. DOI: 10.1186/1471-2458-6-169.

[11] Jessor R, Jessor S. Problem behaviour and psychosocial development: A longitudinal study of youth. New York: Academic press, 1997.

[12] Balogun O, Koyanagi A, Stickley A, Gilmour S, Shibuya K. Alcohol consumption and psychological distress in adolescents: A multi-country study. J Adolesc Health 2014;54(2): 228-34.

[13] Pengpid S, Peltzer K. Alcohol use and misuse among school-going adolescents in Laos: Investigating socio-ecological factors. Int J Child Adolesc Health 2019;12(2):197-204.

[14] Peltzer K, Pengpid S, Tepirou C. Associations of alcohol use with mental health and alcohol exposure among school-going students in Cambodia. Nagoya J Med Sci 2016;78(4):415-22. doi: 10.18999/nagjms.78.4.415.

[15] Reid SD. Time for a regional alcohol policy - A literature review of the burden of normative alcohol use in the Caribbean. J Public Health Policy 2015;36(4):469-83. doi: 10.1057/jphp.2015.27.

[16] Das JK, Salam RA, Arshad A, Finkelstein Y, Bhutta ZA. Interventions for adolescent substance abuse: An overview of systematic reviews. J Adolesc Health 2016:59(4S):S61-S75. doi: 10.1016/j.jadohealth.2016.06.021.

In: Adolescence in Curaçao
Editors: Soraya Verstraeten et al.
ISBN: 978-1-53617-522-6

Chapter 10

PREVALENCE AND PREDICTORS OF SHORT SLEEP AMONG A NATIONALLY REPRESENTATIVE SAMPLE OF SCHOOL-GOING ADOLESCENTS IN CURAÇAO

Karl Peltzer*[1], *PhD*, *Supa Pengpid*[1,2,*], *DrPH* and *Soraya Verstraeten*[3], *MA

[1]Department of Research Administration and Development, University of Limpopo, Turfloop, South Africa

[2]ASEAN Institute for Health Development, Mahidol University, Salaya, Phutthamonthon, Nakhon Pathom, Thailand

[3]Institute for Public Health (Volksgezondheid Instituut Curaçao), Ministry of Public Health, Environment and Nature, Willemstad, Curaçao

[*] ***Correspondence***: Professor Supa Pengpid, ASEAN Institute for Health Development, Mahidol University, 25/25 Phutthamonthon Road 4, Salaya, Phutthamonton, Nakhon Pathom 73170, Thailand. E-Mail: supaprom@yahoo.com.

ABSTRACT

In this chapter we assess the prevalence and correlates of short sleep among a national sample of in-school adolescents in Curaçao. In the cross-sectional Curaçao "Global School-Based Student Health Survey (GSHS)" in 2015, 2,765 adolescents (median age 15 years) responded to questions on sociodemographic, internal, external and socio-familial factors and sleep duration. The prevalence of school night short sleep was 63.3%. The average sleep duration decreased from 7.68 hours at age 11 or 12 years to 6.62 hours at 18 years of age. In adjusted logistic regression analysis, multiple psychological distress (Adjusted Odds Ratio-AOR: 1.51, 95% Confidence Interval-CI: 1.08-2.11) and skipping breakfast (AOR: 1.45, 95% CI: 1.17-1.80) were positively, and older age (17 years and older) (AOR: 0.67. 95% CI: 0.53-0.85), male sex (AOR: 0.76, 95% CI: 0.61-0.95), and high parental support (AOR: 0.72, 95% CI: 0.53-0.97) were negatively associated with short sleep. A high prevalence and several factors associated with short sleep were identified, which can guide in the development of interventions.

INTRODUCTION

"Adequate sleep contributes to a student's overall health and well-being." (1) The National Sleep Foundation (2) recommends "9-11 hours for 6-13 year-old children, 8-10 hours for 14-17 year-olds and 7-9 hours for 18-25 year-olds for optimal health." In a national US survey, the majority of high school students (72.7%) had insufficient sleep (<8 hours for 13-18 year olds) on school nights (3), and in a study among 15-17 year-olds in Norway, 32.3% reported short sleep (<8 h/day) on school nights (4). The prevalence of short sleep duration (<8 h on school days) among adolescents (10-19 years) in Brazil was 53.6% (5), in China 40% (13-18 years) (6) and in Kuwait (aged 14-19 years), 76% of boys and 74% of girls in Kuwait had short sleep (<7 h/day) (7). Among university students in the Caribbean, the prevalence of short sleep (<7 h/day) was 51.4% in Barbados, 45.8% in Grenada, and 55.8% in Jamaica (8). There is lack of studies investigating the prevalence of short sleep and its correlates among adolescents in the Caribbean.

It is important to identify possible risk factors for short sleep among adolescents in order to better design appropriate interventions. Previous studies identified sociodemographic, internal factors, external factors and socio-familial factors associated with short sleep among adolescents. Sociodemographic factors associated with short sleep among adolescents may include older age (5, 9) and low socioeconomic status (10, 11). Internal factors associated with short sleep among adolescents may include poor health status, poor mental health status (12), depression (9) and religious involvement (13).

External factors increasing the odds for short sleep among adolescents may include school shift (5), early school start times (14), extracurricular activities (14), excessive homework load (14), physical inactivity (8, 15, 16), sedentary behaviour (16,17), use of electronic media (14), problematic Internet use (9), tobacco and alcohol use (18,19), marijuana use (19), caffeine intake (9,14), skipping breakfast (7), and intake of fast foods and sugar-sweetened drinks (7). In addition, physical inactivity (8, 15, 16) and sedentary behaviour (16, 17) increased the odds for short sleep. Socio-familial factors associated with short sleep among adolescents may include time spent with peers (20), negative family environment (9, 18) and lack of parental monitoring of adolescents (21). Studies on short sleep and its correlates among adolescents have predominantly been conducted in North America and Europe, and less is known about this in the Caribbean, such as in Curaçao. The study aimed to assess the prevalence and correlates of short sleep among a nationally representative sample of school-going adolescents in Curaçao.

OUR STUDY

Cross-sectional data from the 2015 Curaçao GSHS were analyzed (22). The study used a two-stage cluster sample design to produce data representative of all students enrolled in public secondary education, comparable to US Grades 1-6, in Curaçao. "At the first stage, 28 schools were selected with probability proportional to enrollment size, and at the second stage, 161 classes were randomly selected" (23). All students in selected classes were eligible to participate after ethical approval *in accordance with the "WMA Declaration of Helsinki – Ethical Principles for Medical Research Involving Human Subjects"* and other permissions were granted and written informed consent was obtained from parents and children; the overall response rate was 83% (23).

Measures

The GSHS questionnaire applied to this analysis was used in this survey (see Appendix 1) (24). Sleep duration was assessed with the question, "On an average school night, how many hours of sleep do you get?" (Response options ranged from four or less hours to 10 or more hours). Following recommendations of the "National Sleep Foundation" (2), "normal sleep duration for optimal health was defined as 9-11 hours for 6-13 year-old children, 8-10 hours for 14-17 year-olds and 7-9 hours for 18-25 year-olds." Short sleep was defined as less than the normal or recommended sleep duration. "Inadequate fruit and vegetable consumption was classified as less than five servings per day" (25). "Inadequate physical activity was defined as not daily at least 60 minutes of moderate to vigorous-intensity physical activity" (26). Sedentary behaviour was defined as "spending 3 or more hours per day sitting" (27). The four parental support items were combined and grouped into 0-1 low, 2 medium and 3-4 high support. Psychological distress was defined as zero, single as one and multiple as 2-5 psychological distress items (anxiety, loneliness, no close friends, suicidal ideation and suicide attempt).

Data analysis

Data analysis was conducted with "STATA software version 15.0 (Stata Corporation, College Station, TX, USA)", considering the complex study design. Multivariable logistic regression was used to assess the associations between independent variables (sociodemographic, internal, external and socio-familial factors) and short sleep; variables found significant in bivariate analyses were subsequently included into the multivariable model. Missing data were excluded from the analysis. P values <0.05 were considered significant.

FINDINGS

The sample consisted of 2,765 school-going adolescents (median age 15 years, interquartile range 3), 51.1% female and 48.9% male, 3.8% had mostly or always experienced hunger in the past month, and 81.7% had parents or guardians that provided them mostly or always with necessities. The prevalence of short sleep was 63.3%. The prevalence of the assessed internal, external and socio-familial factors are described in Table 1.

Figure 1 shows the decreasing trend in sleep duration from 7.68 hours at age 11 or 12 years to 6.62 hours at 18 years of age (see Figure 1). Figure 2 shows the prevalence of short sleep by age and sex, which was the lowest at age 18 years (47.3%), followed by 14 year-olds (55.0%), and was the highest at ages 13 years (77.4%) and 17 years (76.8%) (see Figure 2).

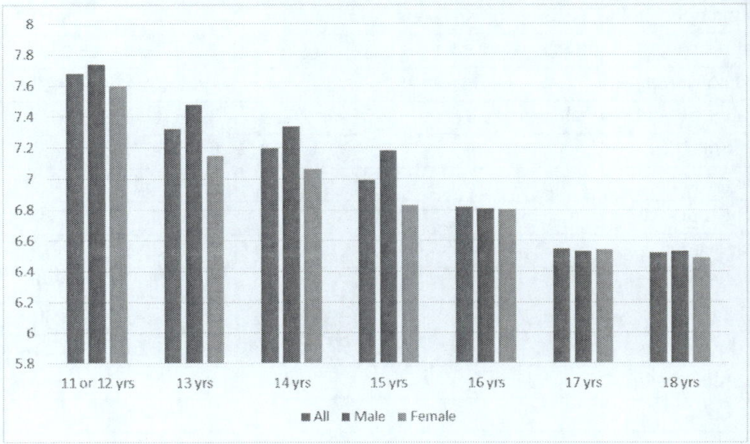

Figure 1. School night sleep duration in hours by age and sex.

Table 1. Sample and short sleep characteristics

Variables	Sample	Short sleep
Sociodemographic factors	N (%)	%
All	2765	63.3
Age in years		
≤11-14	1054 (32.8)	64.8
15-16	824 (32.7)	65.6
17-18 or more	877 (34.5)	59.7
Sex		
Female	1508 (51.1)	65.7
Male	1230 (48.9)	60.6
Hunger	102 (3.8)	67.3
Parents provide necessities	2082 (81.7)	62.3
Internal factors		
Psychological distress		
None	1719 (65.1)	61.4
Single	531 (20.5)	61.7
Multiple	379 (14.4)	75.1
Religious or spiritual person	1717 (69.0)	61.5
External factors		
Physical inactivity	2317 (88.2)	63.4
Sedentary behaviour	1613 (61.9)	63.7
Current tobacco use	345 (13.2)	70.3
Heavy alcohol use	477 (19.0)	68.0
Current cannabis use	136 (5.7)	73.3
Used methamphetamine, cocaine, or XTC one or more times	45 (1.7)	89.0
Daily soft drink consumption	1670 (60.9)	64.4
Fast food consumption	1903 (69.0)	62.9
Inadequate fruit and vegetable intake	2263 (83.5)	64.3
Skipping breakfast	949 (34.7)	68.3
In physical fight	492 (17.9)	70.5
Physically attacked	394 (14.3)	73.0
Carried a weapon	363 (13.9)	71.5
Belong to violent gang	165 (6.1)	66.1
Was bullied	683 (25.4)	68.0
Perceived overweight	787 (28.6)	67.4
Socio-familial factors		
Peer support	1241 (47.6)	61.7

Variables	Sample	Short sleep
Parental support		
Low	665 (27.2)	70.0
Medium	659 (26.7)	63.1
High	1167 (46.1)	59.4
Lives with both parents	1325 (48.9)	63.4
No adult to rely on with personal problems	499 (18.5)	63.8
Experienced physical violence from parents	417 (15.2)	69.1

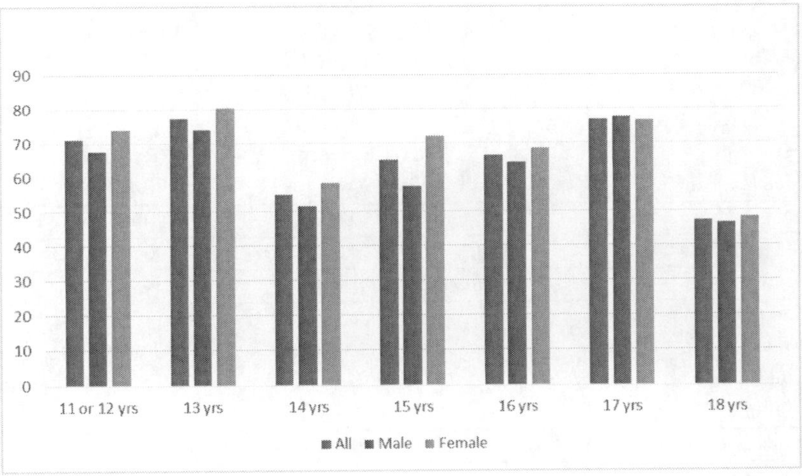

Figure 2. Prevalence of short sleep in percent by age and sex.

Associations with short sleep

In adjusted logistic regression analysis, multiple psychological distress (Adjusted Odds Ratio-AOR: 1.51, 95% Confidence Interval-CI: 1.08-2.11) and skipping breakfast (AOR: 1.45, 95% CI: 1.17-1.80) were positively, and older age (17 years and older) (AOR: 0.67. 95% CI: 0.53-0.85), male sex (AOR: 0.76, 95% CI: 0.61-0.95), and high parental support (AOR: 0.72, 95% CI: 0.53-0.97) were negatively associated with short sleep. In addition, in unadjusted analysis, the parental provision of necessities was inversely associated with short sleep, and substance use (tobacco, alcohol, cannabis, methamphetamine and other drugs), violence (in physical fight, physically attacked, carried a weapon, belonged to a violent group and was bullied), perceived overweight and experienced physical violence from parents were positively associated with short sleep (see Table 2).

Table 2. Associations with short sleep

	UOR (95% CI)	AOR (95% CI)
Sociodemographic factors		
Age in years		
≤11-14	1 (Reference)	1 (Reference)
15-16	1.04 (0.86, 1.25)	0.95 (0.76, 1.18)
17-18 or more	0.81 (0.65, 0.99)*	0.67 (0.53, 0.85)**
Sex		
Female	1 (Reference)	1 (Reference)
Male	0.80 (0.66, 0.97)*	0.76 (0.61, 0.95)*
Hunger	1.20 (0.66, 2.18)	---
Parents provide necessities	0.81 (0.66, 0.99)*	1.06 (0.83, 1.35)
Internal factors		
Psychological distress		
None	1 (Reference)	1 (Reference)
Single	101 (0.78, 1.31)	0.90 (0.66, 1.23)
Multiple	1.90 (1.44, 2.51)***	1.51 (1.08, 2.11)*
Religious or spiritual person	0.85 (0.69, 1.04)	---
External factors		
Physical inactivity	1.00 (0.81, 1.24)	---
Sedentary behaviour	1.03 (0.82, 1.29)	---
Current tobacco use	1.44 (1.12, 1.84)**	0.98 (0.69, 1.30)
Heavy alcohol use	1.28 (1.02, 1.62)*	1.28 (0.97, 1.68)
Current cannabis use	1.64 (1.12, 2.40)*	1.10 (0.70, 1.74)
Other drugs	4.77 (1.73, 13.18)**	2.93 (0.64, 13.31)
Daily soft drink consumption	1.14 (0.98, 1.33)	---
Fast food consumption	0.96 (0.81, 1.14)	---
Inadequate fruit and vegetable intake	1.29 (0.99, 1.72)	---
Skipping breakfast	1.39 (1.17, 1.66)***	1.45 (1.17, 1.80)***
In physical fight	1.47 (1.10, 1.95)**	1.18 (0.83, 1.68)
Physically attacked	1.67 (1.22, 2.28)**	1.28 (0.94, 1.76)
Carried a weapon	1.52 (1.13, 2.04)**	1.31 (0.88, 1.95)
Belong to violent group	1.15 (0.78, 1.70)	---
Was bullied	1.33 (1/08, 1.63)**	1.08 (0.83, 1.41)
Perceived overweight	1.30 (1.07, 1.59)**	1.26 (0.99, 1.59)

	UOR (95% CI)	AOR (95% CI)
Socio-familial factors		
Peer support	0.88 (0.74, 1.04)	---
Parental support		
Low	1 (Reference)	1 (Reference)
Medium	0.73 (0.60, 0.92)*	0.83 (0.62, 1.11)
High	0.63 (0.49, 0.81)***	0.72 (0.53, 0.97)*
Lives with both parents	1.00 (0.86, 1.16)	---
No adult to rely on with personal problems	1.03 (0.82, 1.29)	---
Experienced physical violence from parents	1.36 (1.06, 1.73)*	1.02 (0.76, 1.37)

UOR = Unadjusted Odd Ratio, AOR = Adjusted Odds Ratio; ***P < 0.001, **P < 0.01. *P < 0.05.

DISCUSSION

The study found in a national sample of school-going adolescents in Curaçao a high prevalence of school night short sleep (63.3%), which seems lower than among high school students in the USA (72.7%) (3) and Kuwait (75%) (7), but higher than in other studies among adolescents in Brazil (53.6%) (5), in China (40%) (6), in Norway (32.3%) (4), and among university students in Barbados (51.4%), Grenada (45.8%) and Jamaica (55.8%) (8). Some of these differences between countries may be attributed to different cut-off definitions of short sleep and to different age distributions within the study populations.

Consistent with previous studies (5, 9), this study found that sleep duration reduced with age, but short sleep decreased with age. The latter may be explained by the new National sleep foundation guideline that classified 18 years and older students with <7 hours as short sleep, while previously and other studies used a cut-off definition of <8 hours for short sleep for this age group. According to Owens and Weiss (14) short sleep in the adolescent period may be attributed "internal biological processes such as the normal shift (delay) in circadian rhythm that occurs in association with puberty and a developmentally-based slowing of the sleep drive."

Some studies found that low socioeconomic status (10, 11) was associated with short sleep, while in this study in bivariate analysis the lack of parental provision of necessities was associated with short sleep, but the experience of hunger (as a proxy for socioeconomic status) was not associated with short sleep. While some previous studies (5, 8, 9) did not find significant gender differences in the prevalence of short sleep, this study found a significantly higher prevalence of short sleep among girls than boys did. In line with this result, psychological distress, including anxiety, loneliness, suicide ideation and suicide attempt, was also more prevalent among girls in Curaçao (23).

In agreement with previous studies (9, 12), this study found that psychological distress, including loneliness, anxiety, suicide ideation and suicide attempt, was associated with short sleep. This study did not find that being a religious or spiritual person was protective from short sleep, as found in a previous study (13).

From various external factors analysed, only skipping breakfast remained in adjusted analysis significantly associated with short sleep, which was also identified in a previous investigation among adolescents in Kuwait (7). Previous studies (18, 19) found an association between substance use (alcohol, tobacco, cannabis) and short sleep, while in this study such associations were only found in the unadjusted analysis. Contrary to some previous studies (15-17) among adolescents, this study did not find an association between sedentary behaviour or physical inactivity and short sleep. Some other studies (e.g., 28) did also not find an association between overall physical inactivity and sedentary time and short sleep but found associations with increased screen time. Therefore, it would be important assess sedentary behaviour in terms of screen and non-screen time domains in order to estimate possible effects of screen time on short sleep.

The investigation found that high parental support was protective from short sleep and in unadjusted analysis, negative family environment (experience of physical violence from parents) was associated with short sleep. These findings are in agreement with previous findings (9, 18, 21). This could possibly mean that improving the family environment and increasing parental monitoring of adolescents may be beneficial in increasing sleep duration.

STUDY LIMITATIONS

The study was cross-sectional, so no causal conclusions can be drawn between sleep duration, health risk behaviours and mental health outcomes. The measures utilized in this study were based on self-reports, e.g., sleep duration, physical activity and sedentary behaviours. In future studies more elaborate measuring instruments with objective verification should be used. Sleep duration was only assessed for school days and not for weekends. Future studies should assess sleep duration at both school days and weekend days. Certain external factors, such as school shift, early school start times, extracurricular activities, excessive homework load, screen time or electronic media use, that were previously found relevant for sleep quantity (5, 9, 14) were not assessed in this study should be included in future investigations.

CONCLUSION

The study showed a high prevalence of short sleep among school-going adolescents in Curaçao and identified several associated factors, such as female sex, psychological distress, skipping breakfast and lack of parental support, which should be taken into account in sleep health promotion programmes in this adolescent population.

APPENDIX 1. DESCRIPTION OF VARIABLES USED IN THIS STUDY

Variables	Question	Response options (Coding scheme)
Sleep duration	"On an average school night, how many hours of sleep do you get?"	"1 = 4 or less hours to 7 = 10 or more hours)"
	Sociodemographic factors	
Age	"How old are you?"	"11 years old or younger to 18 years old or older"
Sex	"What is your sex?"	"Male, Female"
Hunger	"During the past 30 days, how often did you go hungry because there was not enough food in your home?"	"1 = never to 5 = always (coded 1–3 = 0 and 4–5 = 1)"
Provision of necessities	"During the past 30 days, how often did your parents or guardians provide for your necessities?"	"1 = never to 5 = always (coded 1–3 = 0 and 4–5 = 1)"
	Internal factors	
	Psychological distress	
No close friends	"How many close friends do you have?"	"1 = 0 to 4 = 3 or more (coded 1+ = 0, 0 = 1)"
Anxiety	"During the past 12 months, how often have you been so worried about something that you could not sleep at night?"	"1 = never to 5 = always (coded 1–3 = 0 and 4–5 = 1)"
Loneliness	"During the past 12 months, how often have you felt lonely?"	"1 = never to 5 = always (coded 1–3 = 0 and 4–5 = 1)"
Suicide ideation	"During the past 12 months, did you ever seriously consider attempting suicide?"	"Yes, No"
Suicide attempt	"During the past 12 months, how many times did you actually attempt suicide?"	"1 = 0 times to 5 = 6 or more times (coded 1 = 0 and 2–5 = 1)"

Variables	Question	Response options (Coding scheme)
	Religiosity	
Religious or spiritual person	"Do you think of yourself as a religious or spiritual person?"	"Yes, No"
	External factors	
Physical activity	"Physical activity is any activity that increases your heart rate and makes you get out of breath some of the time. Physical activity can be done in sports, playing with friends, or walking to school. Some examples of physical activity are running, fast walking, biking, dancing, football, swimming, baseball, and cross-fit. During the past 7 days, on how many days were you physically active for a total of at least 60 minutes per day?"	"0 = 0 days to 7 = 7 days (coded 0 = 0 and 1-7 = 1)"
Leisure-time sedentary behaviour	"How much time do you spend during a typical or usual day sitting and watching television, playing computer games, talking with friends, or doing other sitting activities, such as main play station?"	"1 = Less than 1 hour per day… 3 = 3 to 4 hours per day …6 = 8 or more hours a day" (coded 3 or more hours/day)
Current tobacco use	"During the past 30 days, on how many days did you smoke cigarettes/use any tobacco products other than cigarettes, such as cigars, cigarillos, or electronic cigarettes?"	"1 = 0 days to 7 = All 30 days (coded 1 = 0 and 2-7 = 1)"
Heavy alcohol use (2 or more/day)	"During the past 30 days, on the days you drink alcohol, how many drinks did you usually drink per day?"	1 = Not drink in the past 30 days to 7 = 5 or more drinks (coded 1–3 = 0 and 4–7 = 1)
Current cannabis use	"During the past 30 days, how many times have you used marijuana (also called weed, pot, cannabis, ganja, or grass)?"	"1 = 0 days to 7 = All 30 days (coded 1 = 0 and 2-7 = 1)"
Lifetime methamphetamine, etc. use	"During your life, how many times have you used methamphetamine, cocaine, or XTC (also called speed, base, rock, crack, and uppers)?"	1 = 0 times to 5 = 20 or more times (coded 1 = 0 and 2-5 = 1)

Appendix 1. (Continued)

Variables	Question	Response options (Coding scheme)
	External factors	
Soft drink consumption	"During the past 30 days, how many times per day did you usually drink carbonated soft drinks, such as Coke, Sprite, fria, monster, busta, RedBull, coco rico, and malta? (Do not include diet soft drinks.)"	1 = I did not drink carbonated soft drinks during the past 30 days to 7 = 5 or more times per day (coded 1 = once or more/day)
Fast food consumption	"During the past 7 days, on how many days did you eat food from a fast food restaurant, such as McDonalds, KFC, Burger King, Pizza Hut, or Wendy's?"	"0 = 0 days to 7 = 7 days (coded 0 = 0 and 1-7 = 1)"
Fruits	"During the past 30 days, how many times per day did you usually eat fruit such as papaya, melon, banana, apples, grape, or pineapple?"	"1 = I did not eat fruit during the past 30 days to 7 = 5 or more times per day"
Vegetables	"During the past 30 days, how many times per day did you usually eat vegetables, such as carrots, beans, tomato, cabbage, or pumpkin?"	"I did not eat vegetables during the past 30 days to 7 = 5 or more times per day "
Skipping breakfast	"During the past 30 days, how often did you eat breakfast?"	"1 = never to 5 = always (coded 1-3 = 1 and 4-5 = 0)
In a physical fight	"During the past 12 months, how many times were you in a physical fight?"	"1 = 0 times to 8 = 12 or more times (coded 1 = 0 and 2–8 = 1)"
Physically attacked	"During the past 12 months, how many times were you physically attacked?"	"1 = 0 times to 8 = 12 or more times (coded 1 = 0 and 2–8 = 1)"
Carried a weapon	"During the past 30 days, on how many days did you carry a weapon, such as a gun, knife, club, or brass knuckles?"	1 = 0 days to 5 = 6 or more days) (coded 1 = 0 and 2-6 = 1)
Belong to violent group	"Do you belong to any violent group?"	"Yes, No"

Variables	Question	Response options (Coding scheme)
	External factors	
Bullied	"During the past 30 days, on how many days were you bullied?"	"1 = 0 days to 7 = All 30 days (coded 1 = 0 and 2–7 = 1)"
Perceived body weight	"How do you describe your weight?"	1 = very underweight to 5 = very overweight) (coded 1-2 = underweight, 3 = normal, 4-5 overweight)
	Socio-familial factors	
Peer support	"During the past 30 days, how often were most of the students in your school kind and helpful?"	"1 = never to 5 = always (coded 1–3 = 0 and 4–5 = 1)"
Parental supervision	"During the past 30 days, how often did your parents or guardians check to see if your homework was done?"	"1 = never to 5 = always (coded 1–3 = 0 and 4–5 = 1)"
Parental connectedness	"During the past 30 days, how often did your parents or guardians understand your problems and worries?"	"1 = never to 5 = always (coded 1–3 = 0 and 4–5 = 1)"
Parental bonding	"During the past 30 days, how often did your parents or guardians really know what you were doing with your free time?	"1 = never to 5 = always (coded 1–3 = 0 and 4–5 = 1)"
Parental respect for privacy	"During the past 30 days, how often did your parents or guardians go through your things without your approval?"	"1 = never to 5 = always (coded 1–3 = 0 and 4–5 = 1)"
Lives with both parents	"Which adult family members do you live with?"	1 = both my mother and father to 5 = I do not live with any adult family members (coded 2-5 = 0 and 1 = 1)
No adult to rely on	"How many adults can you rely on when you have personal problems?"	"1 = 0 to 4 = 3 or more (coded 1+ = 0, 0 = 1)"
Physical violence from parents	"During the past 12 months, did your parents or guardians ever hit, slap, or physically hurt you on purpose?"	"Yes, No"

References

[1] Centers for Disease Control and Prevention (CDC) Sleep and health, 2018. URL: https://www.cdc.gov/healthyschools/sleep.htm.

[2] National sleep foundation. National sleep foundation recommends new sleep times, 2019. URL: https://www.sleepfoundation.org/press-release/national-sleep-foundation-recommends-new-sleep-times/page/0/1.

[3] Wheaton AG, Everett Jones S, Cooper AC, Croft JB. Short sleep duration among middle school and high school students — United States, 2015. *MMWR 2018;*67:85–90.

[4] Stea TH, Knutsen T, Torstveit MK. Association between short time in bed, health-risk behaviors and poor academic achievement among Norwegian adolescents. Sleep Med 2014;15(6):666-71. doi: 10.1016/j.sleep.2014.01.019.

[5] Felden ÉP, Filipin D, Barbosa DG, Andrade RD, Meyer C, Louzada FM. Factors associated with short sleep duration in adolescents. Rev Paul Pediatr 2016;34(1):64-70. doi: 10.1016/j.rpped.2015.05.006.

[6] Gong QH, Li H, Zhang XH, Zhang T, Cui J, Xu GZ. Associations between sleep duration and physical activity and dietary behaviors in Chinese adolescents: results from the Youth Behavioral Risk Factor Surveys of 2015. Sleep Med 2017;37:168-173. doi: 10.1016/j.sleep.2017.06.024.

[7] Al-Haifi AA, AlMajed HT, Al-Hazzaa HM, Musaiger AO, Arab MA, Hasan RA. Relative contribution of obesity, sedentary behaviors and dietary habits to sleep duration among Kuwaiti Adolescents. Glob J Health Sci 2015;8(1):107-17. doi: 10.5539/gjhs.v8n1p107.

[8] Peltzer K, Pengpid S. Sleep duration and health correlates among university students in 26 countries. Psychol Health Med 2016;21:2:208-20, doi:10.1080/13548506.2014.998687

[9] Yen CF, Ko CH, Yen JY, Cheng CP. The multidimensional correlates associated with short nocturnal sleep duration and subjective insomnia among Taiwanese adolescents. Sleep 2008;31(11):1515-25.

[10] BaHammam A, Bin Saeed A, Al-Faris E, Shaikh S. Sleep duration and its correlates in a sample of Saudi elementary school children. Singapore Med J 2006;47:875-81.

[11] Dorofaeff TF, Denny S. Sleep and adolescence. Do New Zealand teenagers get enough? J Paediatr Child Health 2006;42:515-20.

[12] Kaneita Y, Ohida T, Osaki Y, Tanihata T, Minowa M, Suzuki K, et al. Association between mental health status and sleep status among adolescents in Japan: a nationwide cross-sectional survey. J Clin Psychiatry 2007;68(9):1426-35.

[13] Hill TD, Deangelis R, Ellison CG. Religious involvement as a social determinant of sleep: an initial review and conceptual model. Sleep Health 2018;4(4):325-30. doi: 10.1016/j.sleh.2018.04.001.

[14] Owens JA, Weiss MR. Insufficient sleep in adolescents: causes and consequences. Minerva Pediatr 2017;69(4):326-36. doi: 10.23736/S0026-4946.17.04914-3.

[15] Al-Hazzaa HM, Musaiger AO, Abahussain NA, Al-Sobayel HI, Qahwaji DM. Lifestyle correlates of self-reported sleep duration among Saudi adolescents: a multicentre school-based cross-sectional study. Child Care Health Dev 2014;40(4):533-42. doi: 10.1111/cch.12051.

[16] Kim Y, Umeda M, Lochbaum M, Stegemeier S. Physical activity, screen-based sedentary behavior, and sleep duration in adolescents: Youth Risk Behavior Survey, 2011-2013. Prev Chronic Dis 2016;13:E131. doi: 10.5888/pcd13.160245.

[17] Choi H, Kim C, Ko H, Park CG. Relationship between sedentary time and sleep duration among Korean adolescents. J School Nurs 2019. doi: 10.1177/1059840519842230.

[18] Bartel KA, Gradisar M, Williamson P. Protective and risk factors for adolescent sleep: a meta-analytic review. Sleep Med Rev 2015;21:72-85. doi: 10.1016/j.smrv.2014.08.002.

[19] Kwon M, Park E, Dickerson SS. Adolescent substance use and its association to sleep disturbances: A systematic review. Sleep Health 2019;5(4):382-94. doi: 10.1016/j.sleh.2019.06.001.

[20] Mednick SC, Christakis NA, Fowler JH. The spread of sleep loss influences drug use in adolescent social networks. PLoS One 2010;5:e9775.

[21] Gunn HE, O'Rourke F, Dahl RE, Goldstein TR, Rofey DL, Forbes EE, Shaw DS. Young adolescent sleep is associated with parental monitoring. Sleep Health 2019;5(1):58-63. doi: 10.1016/j.sleh.2018.09.001.

[22] World Health Organization (WHO). Global School-based Student Health Survey. Curacao 2015 fact sheet. URL: https://www.who.int/ncds/surveillance/gshs/2015_Curacao_GSHS_Fact_Sheet.pdf.

[23] Verstraeten S. National report the Curaçao Global School-based Student Health Survey (GSHS) study 2015. URL: https://www.who.int/ncds/surveillance/gshs/Final_report_2015_GSHS_Curacao.pdf.

[24] World Health Organization (WHO). Global School-based Student Health Survey (GSHS). 2015 Curacao GSHS Questionnaire. URL: https://www.who.int/ncds/surveillance/gshs/2015_GSHS_Curacao_Questionnaire.pdf.

[25] World Health Organization (WHO). Diet, nutrition and the prevention of chronic diseases. Geneva, Switzerland: WHO, 2003.

[26] World Health Organization (WHO). Physical activity fact sheet, 2017. URL: http://www.who.int/mediacentre/factsheets/fs385/en/.

[27] Guthold R, Cowan MJ, Autenrieth CS, Kann L, Riley LM. Physical activity and sedentary behavior among schoolchildren: a 34-country comparison. J Pediatrics 2010;157:43-9.

[28] Kakinami L, O'Loughlin EK, Brunet J, Dugas EN, Constantin E, Sabiston CM, et al. Associations between physical activity and sedentary behavior with sleep quality and quantity in young adults. Sleep Health 2017;3(1):56-61. doi: 10.1016/j.sleh. 2016.11.001.

In: Adolescence in Curaçao
Editors: Soraya Verstraeten et al.
ISBN: 978-1-53617-522-6

Chapter 11

SHORT SLEEP DURATION AND HEALTH RISK BEHAVIOURS AMONG IN-SCHOOL ADOLESCENTS IN CURAÇAO: RESULTS FROM A NATIONAL CROSS-SECTIONAL SURVEY

Supa Pengpid[1,2,*], DrPH, Soraya Verstraeten[3], MSc and Karl Peltzer[3], PhD

[1]ASEAN Institute for Health Development,
Mahidol University, Salaya, Phutthamonthon,
Nakhon Pathom, Thailand

[2]Department of Research Administration and Development,
University of Limpopo, Turfloop, South Africa

[3]Institute for Public Health (Volksgezondheid Instituut Curaçao),
Ministry of Public Health, Environment and Nature,
Willemstad, Curaçao

---

* ***Correspondence***: Professor Supa Pengpid, ASEAN Institute for Health Development, Mahidol University, 25/25 Phutthamonthon Road 4, Salaya, Phutthamonton, Nakhon Pathom 73170, Thailand. E-Mail: supaprom@yahoo.com.

Abstract

Short sleep may negatively affect health behaviour. We aimed to assess the associations between short sleep and health risk behaviours among a nationally representative sample of school adolescents in Curaçao. In the cross-sectional Curaçao "Global School-Based Student Health Survey (GSHS)" in 2015, 2,765 adolescents (median age 15 years) responded to questions on sleep duration and health risk behaviours. The prevalence of normal sleep was 26.7%, short sleep 46.5% and very short sleep 16.8% during school nights, using National Sleep Foundation recommendations. In adjusted logistic regression analysis, short and/or very short sleep was associated with poor mental health, substance use, perceived overweight, violent or delinquent behaviour, transportation risk-taking and poor hand hygiene behaviours. Short sleep was associated with various health risk behaviours, warranting a response with measures to reduce the burden of sleep loss in this adolescent population.

Introduction

"Adequate sleep contributes to a student's overall health and well-being. Children and adolescents who do not get enough sleep have a higher risk for physical and mental health problems" (1, 2). The "National Sleep Foundation" (3) recommends "9-11 hours for 6-13 year-old children, 8-10 hours for 14-17 year-olds and 7-9 hours for 18-25 year-olds for optimal health." In a national US survey, the majority of middle school (57.8%) and high school (72.7%) students had insufficient sleep (<9 hours for children 6-12 years and <8 hours for 13-18 year olds) on school nights (4), and in a study among 15-17 year-olds in Norway, 32.3% reported short sleep (<8 h/day) on school nights (5).

Various studies and systematic reviews found an association between short sleep duration and poor mental health, obesity and health risk behaviours among adolescents. For example, short sleep among adolescents was associated with depression (6), suicidal ideation (7), suicide plan and suicide attempt (8). Short sleep duration among adolescents was associated with childhood obesity (9, 10), underweight (11) and poor weight-related behaviors, such as sugar-sweetened beverage intake (10,12), snack consumption, intake of sweets/candy (5), inadequate fruit and vegetable consumption (10,12), decreased breakfast eating (10),, having an irregular meal pattern (10), and physical inactivity (5, 10).

Health risk behaviours that were linked to short sleep among adolescents include substance use, such as alcohol use (7, 13, 14), smoking (5, 14), drug use (7, 14), cannabis use (13), delinquent or violent behaviour (14), sexual risk-taking (14), transportation related risk-taking (14), injuries (7), and poor academic achievement (5). Studies on sleep duration and health and well-being among adolescents have predominantly been conducted in North America and Europe, and less is known about this relationship in the Caribbean. The study aimed to assess the associations between short sleep and health risk behaviours among a nationally representative sample of in-school adolescents in Curaçao.

OUR STUDY

Cross-sectional data from the 2015 Curaçao GSHS were analyzed (15). The study used a two-stage cluster sampling approach to generate representative data of all students enrolled in public secondary education, comparable to US Grades 1-6, in Curaçao. "At the first stage, 28 schools were selected with probability proportional to enrolment size, and at the second stage, 161 classes were randomly selected" (16). All school students in the selected classes were eligible to participate after ethical approval *in accordance with the "WMA Declaration of Helsinki – Ethical Principles for Medical Research Involving Human Subjects"* and other permissions were granted and informed consent was obtained; the overall response rate was 83% (16).

Measures

The GSHS questionnaire applied to this analysis was used in this survey (see Appendix 1) (17). Sleep duration was assessed with the question, "On an average school night, how many hours of sleep do you get?" (Response options ranged from four or less hours to 10 or more hours). Following recommendations of the National Sleep Foundation (3), "normal sleep duration for optimal health was defined as 9-11 hours for 6-13 year-old children, 8-10 hours for 14-17 year-olds and 7-9 hours for 18-25 year-olds." Short sleep was defined as 1-2 hours less and very short sleep 3 hours less than the normal or recommended sleep duration. "Inadequate fruit and vegetable consumption was classified as less than five servings per day" (18). "Inadequate physical activity was defined as not daily at least 60 minutes of moderate to vigorous-intensity physical activity" (19). Sedentary behaviour was defined as "spending 3 or more hours per day sitting" (20). The four items on parental were grouped and categorized into 0-1 low, 2 medium and 3-4 high support.

Data analysis

Data analysis was conducted with "STATA software version 15.0 (Stata Corporation, College Station, TX, USA)", considering the complex study design. Multivariable logistic regression analyses were used to assess the associations between short sleep categories and each health risk behaviour outcome, adjusted for age, sex, hunger, peer and parental support. Missing data were excluded from the analysis. P values <0.05 were considered significant.

FINDINGS

The sample consisted of 2,765 school-going adolescents (median age 15 years, interquartile range 3 years), 51.1% female and 48.9% male, 3.8% had mostly or always experienced hunger in the past month, and 46.1% reported high parental support and 47.6% high peer support. The prevalence of normal sleep was 26.7%, short sleep 46.5% and very short sleep 16.8%. The prevalence of the assessed health risk behaviours by sleep duration are depicted in Table 1.

Table 1. Sample and sleep duration characteristics

Variable	Sample	Normal sleep	Short sleep	Very short sleep
	N (%)	%	%	%
All	2765	36.7	46.5	16.8
Age in years				
≤13	586 (16.5)	25.3	50.2	24.5
14-17	1648 (63.6)	34.4	47.7	17.9
≥18	521 (19.9)	52.7	39.9	7.4
Sex				
Female	1508 (51.1)	34.3	47.6	18.1
Male	1230 (48.9)	39.4	45.1	15.5
Hunger	102 (3.8)	32.7	41.8	25.5
Peer support	1241 (47.6)	38.3	48.8	12.9
Parental support				
Low (0-1)	665 (27.2)	30.0	46.6	23.4
Medium (2)	659 (26.7)	36.9	47.8	15.4
High (3-4)	1167 (46.1)	40.6	46.1	13.3
Mental health				
Anxiety	306 (11.4)	27.4	47.5	25.1
Loneliness	417 (15.5)	26.9	46.6	26.6
Suicide ideation	308 (11.3)	22.7	52.0	25.3
Suicide plan	247 (9.1)	26.5	48.8	24.7
Suicide attempt	296 (10.8)	30.3	44.9	24.8
Substance use				
Current alcohol use	1028 (40.8)	33.5	47.8	18.8
Current tobacco use	345 (13.2)	29.7	47.4	22.9
Current cannabis use	136 (5.7)	26.7	48.8	24.4
Used methamphetamine, cocaine, or XTC one or more times	45 (1.7)	11.0	50.3	38.7
Body weight and related behaviours				
Perceived overweight	787 (28.6)	32.6	49.6	17.8
Perceived underweight	400 (14.9)	37.8	43.3	18.8
Inadequate fruit and vegetable intake	2263 (83.5)	35.7	48.0	16.4
Skipping breakfast	949 (34.7)	31.7	47.4	20.9
Daily soft drink consumption	1670 (60.9)	35.6	45.5	18.9
Fast food consumption	1903 (69.0)	37.1	46.5	16.4

Table 1. (Continued)

Variable	Sample	Normal sleep	Short sleep	Very short sleep
	N (%)	%	%	%
Sedentary behaviour	1613 (61.9)	36.3	48.5	15.2
Physical inactivity	2317 (88.2)	36.6	46.8	16.6
Other health risk behaviours				
In physical fight	492 (17.9)	29.5	45.3	25.3
Carried a weapon	363 (13.9)	28.5	46.9	24.6
Belong to violent group	165 (6.1)	33.9	39.4	26.7
Was bullied	683 (25.4)	32.0	46.0	22.0
School truancy	652 (26.6)	33.9	44.7	21.4
Not always seatbelt use	1597 (71.9)	33.8	49.1	17.2
Multiple sexual partners	480 (19.5)	36.3	48.5	15.2
Not always wash hands before meals	1862 (68.7)	22.6	49.3	17.1
Not always wash hands after toilet use	888 (33.3)	31.4	51.2	17.3
Not always wash hands with soap	1355 (49.9)	32.2	49.7	18.1

Associations between sleep duration and health risk behaviours

In adjusted logistic regression analysis, short and/or very short sleep were associated with poor mental health (anxiety, loneliness, and suicidal behaviour), substance use (alcohol, tobacco, cannabis, methamphetamine or other drugs), and other health risk behaviours (in physical fight, carried a weapon, belonged to a violent group, was bullied, school truancy, inconsistent seatbelt use, poor hand washing hygiene). Short sleep but not very short sleep was associated with perceived overweight. Short and very short sleep increased the odds for skipping breakfast and very short sleep was associated with daily soft drink intake. Short sleep was not associated with other body weight and related behaviours (underweight, inadequate fruit and vegetable intake, fast food consumption, sedentary behaviour and physical inactivity) (see Table 2).

Table 2. Adjusted associations between short and very short sleep (with normal sleep as reference category) and health risk indicators

Variable	Short sleep	Very short sleep
	AOR (95% CI)1	AOR (95% CI)1
Mental health		
Anxiety	1.40 (1.03, 1.89)*	2.00 (1.26, 3.19)**
Loneliness	1.39 (1.03, 1.87)*	2.14 (1.47, 3.13)***
Suicide ideation	1.85 (1.32, 2.58)***	2.29 (1.54, 3.42)***
Suicide plan	1.45 (1.01, 2.08)*	1.77 (1.07, 2.93)*
Suicide attempt	1.18 (0.83, 1.66)	1.57, 1.08, 2.28)*
Substance use		
Current alcohol use	1.18 (0.98, 1.42)	1.47 (1.10, 1.97)**
Current tobacco use	1.29 (0.95, 1.76)	1.53 (1.07, 2.21)*
Current cannabis use	1.27 (0.79, 2.03)	1.91 (1.22, 3.02)**
Used methamphetamine, cocaine, or XTC one or more times	3.10 (0.93, 10.4)	6.29 (1.85, 21.43)**
Body weight and related behaviours		
Perceived overweight	1.26 (1.01, 1.56)*	1.25 (0.96, 1.64)
Perceived underweight	0.85 (0.63, 1.16)	1.01 (0.71, 1.45)
Inadequate fruit and vegetable intake	1.35 (0.87, 2.07)	1.06 (0.71, 1.59)
Skipping breakfast	1.29 (1.07, 1.56)**	1.60 (1.15, 2.21)**
Daily soft drink consumption	1.03 (0.87, 1.21)	1.55 (1.12, 2.14)**
Fast food consumption	0.98 (0.81, 1.18)	0.92 (0.68, 1.24)
Sedentary behaviour	1.15 (0.91, 1.46)	0.81 (0.61, 1.07)
Physical inactivity	0.98 (0.75, 1.30)	0.71, 0.48, 1.06)
Other health risk behaviours		
In physical fight	1.28 (0.92, 1.78)	1.96 (1.41, 2.73)***
Carried a weapon	1.37 (0.97, 1.93)	2.17 (1.52, 3.10)***
Belong to violent group	0.86 (0.53, 1.41)	1,61 (1.01, 2.57)*
Was bullied	1.21 (0.98, 1.49)	1.53 (1.12, 2.08)**
School truancy	1.07 (0.81, 1.41)	1.59 (1.09, 2.32)*
Not always seatbelt use	1.45 (1.17, 1.79)***	1.84 (1.35, 2.54)***
Multiple sexual partners	1.07 (0.81, 1.42)	1.19 (0.80, 1.79)
Not always wash hands before meals	1.57 (1.21, 2.04)***	1.30 (1.00, 1.70)*
Not always wash hands after toilet use	1.56 (1.23, 1.97)***	1.33 (1.03, 1.73)*
Not always wash hands with soap	1.50 (1.20, 1.87)***	1.49 (1.17, 1.91)**

AOR = Adjusted Odds Ratio; ***P < 0.001; **P < 0.01; *P < 0.05;

[1]Adjusted for age, sex, hunger, peer and parental support.

Discussion

This study focused on assessing the relationship between sleep duration and various health risk indicators in a national sample of school-going adolescents in a Dutch-Caribbean island country, Curaçao. Using the results from self-reported school night sleep duration this study found a high prevalence of insufficient sleep (63.3%), which compares with findings from a national US survey (middle school: 57.8%, and high school: 72.7%) (4), but were higher than in study in Norway (32.3%) (5).

Consistent with previous research findings (6-8), this study found and association between short sleep and poor mental health, including anxiety, loneliness and suicidal behaviour. Some research (9, 10, 21) found that short sleep duration among adolescents was associated with obesity and underweight (11), while this study only found a weak association between short sleep, but not very short sleep, and perceived overweight and no association between short sleep and perceived underweight.

Regarding different weight-related behaviours, this study's findings were in agreement with previous investigations (10,12) that short and/or very short sleep were associated with increased sugar-sweetened beverage consumption and decreased breakfast eating. While other studies (5, 10, 12) also identified associations between short sleep and insufficient fruit and vegetable intake and physical inactivity, this study did not find such associations. Consistent with a number of studies (5, 7, 13, 14), this study found short sleep increased the odds for substance use (alcohol, tobacco, cannabis and other drugs). Nicotine from tobacco use may negatively affect sleep duration, explaining this possible association (22).

Moreover, in agreement with previous research (14), this study found an association between short sleep and violent or delinquent behaviour (in physical fight, carried a weapon, belonged to a violent group, was bullied and school truancy), transport risk-taking and road safety (not always wearing a seatbelt). Unlike in a previous review (14), this study did not find an association between short sleep and sexual risk-taking (multiple sexual partners). In addition, this study found associations between short sleep and poor hand hygiene behaviours. It is possible that according the problem behaviour theory various health risk behaviours are interrelated and cluster together (23).

Some mechanisms have been suggested in order to explain the impact of short sleep on health risk behaviours. For example, "Neuroimaging studies support the notion that sleep duration may impact risk-taking behaviour through its effect on the brain." (14). In this case, adolescents with short sleep may have "dampened reactivity of this reward-related brain region, thus requiring these adolescents to seek more exciting or risky rewards to experience reward circuitry activation."(24) Considering the high prevalence of short sleep and the possible negative effects on a range of health behaviours and mental health outcomes, interventions are warranted, such as school-based sleep education programmes that have previously shown beneficial results (25).

STUDY LIMITATIONS

The current investigation was cross-sectional by design. Therefore, no causal relationship can be established between sleep duration, health risk behaviours and mental health outcomes. The measures utilized in this study were based on self-reports, e.g., sleep duration, physical activity and sedentary behaviours. Future studies may use more elaborate measures with objective verification. The response format of the sleep duration question only allowed assessing "10 or more hours" and not singling hours beyond 10 hours, such as 11 and 12 hours, which hindered us from assessing the associations between health risk behaviours and long sleep duration. In addition, sleep duration was only assessed for school days and not for weekends. Future studies should assess sleep duration at both school days and weekend days.

Conclusion

The study showed a high prevalence of insufficient sleep among school-going adolescents in Curaçao and identified many health risk behaviours associated with an insufficient sleep duration, such as poor mental health, substance use, perceived overweight, violent or delinquent behaviour, transport risk-taking and poor hand hygiene behaviours. In response, school-based policy measures are warranted to reduce the burden of sleep loss on the health of this adolescent population.

Appendix 1. Description and Coding of Variables Used in This Study

Variables	Question	Response options (Coding scheme)
Age	"How old are you?"	"11 years old or younger to 18 years old or older"
Sex	"What is your sex?"	"Male, Female"
Hunger	"During the past 30 days, how often did you go hungry because there was not enough food in your home?"	"1 = never to 5 = always (coded 1–3 = 0 and 4–5 = 1)"
Peer support	"During the past 30 days, how often were most of the students in your school kind and helpful?"	"1 = never to 5 = always (coded 1–3 = 0 and 4–5 = 1)"
Parental supervision	"During the past 30 days, how often did your parents or guardians check to see if your homework was done?"	"1 = never to 5 = always (coded 1–3 = 0 and 4–5 = 1)"
Parental connectedness	"During the past 30 days, how often did your parents or guardians understand your problems and worries?"	"1 = never to 5 = always (coded 1–3 = 0 and 4–5 = 1)"
Parental bonding	"During the past 30 days, how often did your parents or guardians really know what you were doing with your free time?	"1 = never to 5 = always (coded 1–3 = 0 and 4–5 = 1)"
Parental respect for privacy	"During the past 30 days, how often did your parents or guardians go through your things without your approval?"	"1 = never to 5 = always (coded 1–3 = 0 and 4–5 = 1)"

Variables	Question	Response options (Coding scheme)
Sleep duration	"On an average school night, how many hours of sleep do you get?"	"1 = 4 or less hours to 7 = 10 or more hours)"
	Mental health	
Anxiety	"During the past 12 months, how often have you been so worried about something that you could not sleep at night?"	"1 = never to 5 = always (coded 1–3 = 0 and 4–5 = 1)"
Loneliness	"During the past 12 months, how often have you felt lonely?"	"1 = never to 5 = always (coded 1–3 = 0 and 4–5 = 1)"
Suicide ideation	"During the past 12 months, did you ever seriously consider attempting suicide?"	"Yes, No"
Suicide plan	"During the past 12 months, did you make a plan about how you would attempt suicide?"	"Yes, No"
Suicide attempt	"During the past 12 months, how many times did you actually attempt suicide?"	"1 = 0 times to 5 = 6 or more times (coded 1 = 0 and 2–5 = 1)"
	Substance use	
Current alcohol use	"During the past 30 days, on how many days did you have at least one drink containing alcohol?"	"1 = 0 days to 7 = All 30 days (coded 1 = 0 and 2-7 = 1)"
Current tobacco use	"During the past 30 days, on how many days did you smoke cigarettes/use any tobacco products other than cigarettes, such as cigars, cigarillos, or electronic cigarettes?"	"1 = 0 days to 7 = All 30 days (coded 1 = 0 and 2-7 = 1)"
Current cannabis use	"During the past 30 days, how many times have you used marijuana (also called weed, pot, cannabis, ganja, or grass)?"	"1 = 0 days to 7 = All 30 days (coded 1 = 0 and 2-7 = 1)"
Lifetime metham-phetamine, etc. use	"During your life, how many times have you used methamphetamine, cocaine, or XTC (also called speed, base, rock, crack, and uppers)?"	"1 = 0 times to 5 = 20 or more times (coded 1 = 0 and 2-5 = 1)"
	Body weight and related variables	
Perceived body weight	"How do you describe your weight?"	"1 = very underweight to 5 = very overweight) (coded 1-2 = underweight, 3 = normal, 4-5 overweight)"

Appendix 1. (Continued)

Variables	Question	Response options (Coding scheme)
Fruits	"During the past 30 days, how many times per day did you usually eat fruit such as papaya, melon, banana, apples, grape, or pineapple?"	"1 = I did not eat fruit during the past 30 days to 7 = 5 or more times per day"
Vegetables	"During the past 30 days, how many times per day did you usually eat vegetables, such as carrots, beans, tomato, cabbage, or pumpkin?"	"I did not eat vegetables during the past 30 days to 7 = 5 or more times per day "
Skipping breakfast	"During the past 30 days, how often did you eat breakfast?"	1 = never to 5 = always (coded 1-3 = 1 and 4-5 = 0)
Soft drink consumption	"During the past 30 days, how many times per day did you usually drink carbonated soft drinks, such as Coke, Sprite, fria, monster, busta, RedBull, coco rico, and malta? (Do not include diet soft drinks.)"	1 = I did not drink carbonated soft drinks during the past 30 days to 7 = 5 or more times per day (coded 1 = once or more/day)
Fast food consumption	"During the past 7 days, on how many days did you eat food from a fast food restaurant, such as McDonalds, KFC, Burger King, Pizza Hut, or Wendy's?"	"0 = 0 days to 7 = 7 days (coded 0 = 0 and 1-7 = 1)"
Leisure-time sedentary behaviour	"How much time do you spend during a typical or usual day sitting and watching television, playing computer games, talking with friends, or doing other sitting activities, such as main play station?"	"1 = Less than 1 hour per day… 3 = 3 to 4 hours per day …6 = 8 or more hours a day" (coded 3 or more hours/day)
Physical activity	"Physical activity is any activity that increases your heart rate and makes you get out of breath some of the time. Physical activity can be done in sports, playing with friends, or walking to school. Some examples of physical activity are running, fast walking, biking, dancing, football, swimming, baseball, and cross-fit. During the past 7 days, on how many days were you physically active for a total of at least 60 minutes per day?"	"0 = 0 days to 7 = 7 days (coded 0 = 0 and 1-7 = 1)"

Variables	Question	Response options (Coding scheme)
	Other health risk behaviours	
In a physical fight	"During the past 12 months, how many times were you in a physical fight?"	"1 = 0 times to 8 = 12 or more times (coded 1 = 0 and 2–8 = 1)"
Carried a weapon	"During the past 30 days, on how many days did you carry a weapon, such as a gun, knife, club, or brass knuckles?"	1 = 0 days to 5 = 6 or more days) (coded 1 = 0 and 2-6 = 1)
Belong to violent group	"Do you belong to any violent group?"	"Yes, No"
Bullied	"During the past 30 days, on how many days were you bullied?"	"1 = 0 days to 7 = All 30 days (coded 1 = 0 and 2–7 = 1)"
School truancy	"During the past 30 days, on how many days did you miss classes or school without permission?"	"1 = 0 days to 5 = 10 or more days (coded 1 = 1 and 2–5 = 0)"
Seatbelt use	"During the past 30 days, how often did you use a seatbelt when riding in a car or other motor vehicle driven by someone else?"	"1 = not in car to 6 = always) (coded 1 and 6 = 0 and 2-5 = 1)
Multiple sexual partners	"During your life, with how many people have you had sexual intercourse?"	1 = never to 7 = 6 or more people (coded 1-2 = 0 and 3-7 = 1)
Hand washing before eating	"During the past 30 days, how often did you wash your hands before eating?"	"1 = never to 5 = always (coded 1–4 = 1 and 5 = 0)"
Hand washing after toilet	"During the past 30 days, how often did you wash your hands after using the toilet or latrine?"	"1 = never to 5 = always (coded 1–4 = 1 and 5 = 0)"
Using soap when hand washing	"During the past 30 days, how often did you use soap when washing your hands?"	"1 = never to 5 = always (coded 1–4 = 1 and 5 = 0)"

REFERENCES

[1] Chaput JP, Gray CE, Poitras VJ, Carson V, Gruber R, Olds T, et al. Systematic review of the relationships between sleep duration and health indicators in school-aged children and youth. Appl Physiol Nutr Metab 2016;41(6 Suppl 3):S266-82. doi: 10.1139/apnm-2015-0627.

[2] Centers for Disease Control and Prevention (CDC). Sleep and health, 2018. URL: https://www.cdc.gov/healthyschools/sleep.htm

[3] National sleep foundation. National sleep foundation recommends new sleep times, 2019. URL: https://www.sleepfoundation.org/press-release/national-sleep-foundation-recommends-new-sleep-times/page/0/1.

[4] Wheaton AG, Everett Jones S, Cooper AC, Croft JB. Short sleep duration among middle school and high school students — United States, 2015. MMWR 2018;67:85–90.

[5] Stea TH, Knutsen T, Torstveit MK. Association between short time in bed, health-risk behaviors and poor academic achievement among Norwegian adolescents. Sleep Med 2014;15(6):666-71. doi: 10.1016/j.sleep.2014.01.019.

[6] Berger AT, Wahlstrom KL, Widome R. Relationships between sleep duration and adolescent depression: A conceptual replication. Sleep Health 2019;5(2):175-9. doi: 10.1016/j.sleh.2018.12.003.

[7] Owens JA, Weiss MR. Insufficient sleep in adolescents: causes and consequences. Minerva Pediatr 2017;69(4):326-36. doi: 10.23736/S0026-4946.17.04914-3.

[8] Chiu HY, Lee HC, Chen PY, Lai YF, Tu YK. Associations between sleep duration and suicidality in adolescents: A systematic review and dose-response meta-analysis. Sleep Med Rev 2018;42:119-26. doi: 10.1016/j.smrv.2018.07.003.

[9] Li L, Zhang S, Huang Y, Chen K. Sleep duration and obesity in children: A systematic review and meta-analysis of prospective cohort studies. J Paediatr Child Health 2017;53(4):378-385. doi: 10.1111/jpc.13434.

[10] Widome R, Lenk KM, Laska MN, Erickson DJ, Iber C, Kilian G, Wahlstrom K. Sleep duration and weight-related behaviors among adolescents. Child Obes 2019;15(7):434-442. doi: 10.1089/chi.2018.0362.

[11] Pengpid S, Peltzer K. Prevalence of overweight and underweight and its associated factors among male and female university students in Thailand. Homo 2015;66(2):176-86. doi: 10.1016/j.jchb.2014.11.002.

[12] Córdova FV, Barja S, Brockmann PE. Consequences of short sleep duration on the dietary intake in children: A systematic review and metanalysis. Sleep Med Rev 2018;42:68-84. doi: 10.1016/j.smrv.2018.05.006.

[13] Mike TB, Shaw DS, Forbes EE, Sitnick SL, Hasler BP. The hazards of bad sleep duration and quality as predictors of adolescent alcohol and cannabis use. Drug Alcohol Depend 2016;168:335-9. doi: 10.1016/j.drugalcdep.2016.08.009

[14] Short MA, Weber N. Sleep duration and risk-taking in adolescents: A systematic review and meta-analysis. Sleep Med Rev 2018;41:185-96. doi: 10.1016/j.smrv. 2018.03.006.

[15] World Health Organization (WHO). Global School-based Student Health Survey. Curacao 2015 fact sheet. URL: https://www.who.int/ncds/surveillance/gshs/2015_Curacao_GSHS_Fact_Sheet.pdf.

[16] Verstraeten S. National report the Curaçao Global School-based Student Health Survey (GSHS) study 2015. URL: https://www.who.int/ncds/surveillance/gshs/Final_report_2015_GSHS_Curacao.pdf.

include being female (8, 13-15), older adolescents (13-15), low family socioeconomic status (8, 13, 14), and living in single-parent families (13, 14). Body weight status and dietary behaviour for skipping breakfast among adolescents include being underweight (14), overweight/obese, (8, 14, 15), inadequate fruit and vegetable intake (13, 16), consumed less milk (16), soft drink consumption (13), junk food intake (16), and dieting (13, 17).

Substance use factors for skipping breakfast among adolescents include smoking (8, 13) and heavy alcohol use (8, 17). Other health risk behaviour factors for skipping breakfast among adolescents include being physically inactive (8, 13, 14-17), sedentary behaviour (13), long screen time, such as watching TV (15-17), inadequate sleep (14), insufficient sleep (15), and school bullying (18). The study aimed to assess the prevalence and correlates of skipping breakfast among adolescents in Curaçao.

OUR STUDY

Cross-sectional data from the 2015 Curaçao GSHS were analysed (19). The investigation used a two-stage cluster sampling approach to generate representative data of all students enrolled in public secondary education, comparable to US Grades 1-6, in Curaçao. "At the first stage, 28 schools were selected with probability proportional to enrolment size, and at the second stage, 161 classes were randomly selected" (20). All students in selected classes were eligible to participate after ethical approval *in accordance with the "WMA Declaration of Helsinki – Ethical Principles for Medical Research Involving Human Subjects"* and other permissions were granted and informed consent was obtained from parents and children; the overall response rate was 83% (20).

Measures

The GSHS measure was used in this survey (see appendix 1) (19). "Inadequate FV consumption was classified as less than five or more servings in a day" (21, 22). "Inadequate physical activity was defined as not daily at least 60 minutes of moderate to vigorous-intensity physical activity."(23) "Sedentary behaviour was defined as spending three or more hours per day sitting" (24). Short sleep was defined as 1-2 hours less and very short sleep 3 hours less than the normal or recommended sleep duration "defined as 9-11 hours for 6-13 year-old children, 8-10 hours for 14-17 year-olds and 7-9 hours for 18-25 year-olds." (3). "The four items on parental or guardian support were summed, and classified into three groups, 0-1 low, 2 medium and 3-4 high support" (25).

Data analysis

Considering the clustered study design, data analyses were conducted with "STATA software version 15.0 (Stata Corporation, College Station, TX, USA)." Descriptive statistics are used to provide frequencies, means and standard deviations. Unadjusted and adjusted multinomial logistic regression analyses were utilized for assessing the associations between independent variables and two (infrequent and frequent) skipping breakfast categories (with daily or always breakfast as reference category). Data with missing information were excluded from the analyses. P values <0.05% were considered significant.

FINDINGS

The sample consisted of 2,765 school students (median age 15 years, interquartile range 3 years), 51.1% females and 48.9% males, 51.1% were not living with both parents and 81.7% reported parental provision of necessities. Regarding protective indicators, 73.4% of students attended school in the 30 days, 47.6% received frequently support by their peers, 69.0% considered themselves a religious or spiritual person, and 72.8% had two to four parental support scores. In all, 56.9% skipped breakfast (never, rarely, sometimes of most of the time had breakfast) in the past 30 days, 42.2 had sometimes or mostly breakfast and 14.9% had never or rarely had breakfast (see Table 1).

Table 1. Sample and breakfast consumption characteristics

Variable	Sample	Breakfast always (daily)	Breakfast sometimes or mostly	Breakfast never or rarely
	N (%)	%	%	%
	Sociodemographics			
All	2765	43.1	42.2	14.9
Sex				
Female	1508 (51.1)	40.9	44.6	14.5
Male	1230 (48.9)	45.4	39.5	15.2
Age (years)				
≤14	1054 (32.8)	48.0	38.4	13.5
15 or 16	824 (32.7)	41.7	41.6	16.7
≥17	877 (34.5)	39.6	45.8	14.6
Not live with both parents	1384 (51.1)	40.5	43.7	15.9
Parents provide necessities	2082 (81.7)	44.7	41.4	13.9
Body weight and health risk behaviour				
Hungry				
Never or rarely	2379 (86.9)	45.7	41.1	13.2
Sometimes	253 (9.3)	23.8	48.1	28.0
Mostly or always	102 (3.8)	29.7	46.8	23.5
Perceived body weight				
Normal	1521 (56.5)	44.1	42.0	13.8
Underweight	400 (14.9)	40.3	40.3	19.4
Overweight	787 (28.6)	42.0	43.1	15.0
Inadequate fruit and vegetable consumption	2263 (83.5)	41.5	43.5	15.0
Trying to lose weight	1004 (36.2)	42.4	42.5	15.1
Fast food consumption	1903 (69.0)	42.3	43.6	14.1
Soft drink consumption	1670 (60.9)	40.0	44.4	15.7
Current tobacco use	345 (13.2)	36.9	44.5	18.6
Heavy alcohol use	477 (19.0)	41.5	42.3	16.2
Current cannabis use	136 (5.7)	34.7	43.5	21.8

Table 1. (Continued)

Variable	Sample	Breakfast always (daily)	Breakfast sometimes or mostly	Breakfast never or rarely
	N (%)	%	%	%
Sedentary behavior	1613 (61.9)	41.7	43.2	15.1
Physical inactivity	2317 (88.2)	42.0	42.8	15.3
Sleep duration				
Normal	931 (36.7)	48.5	39.5	12.0
Short	1206 (46.5)	41.1	43.7	15.2
Very short	446 (16.8)	37.6	42.2	20.1
Was bullied	683 (25.4)	37.8	43.8	18.4
Protective factors				
School attendance	1976 (73.4)	45.3	40.6	14.1
Peer support	1241 (47.6)	46.1	42.1	11.8
Religious person	1717 (69.0)	45.1	41.3	13.7
Parental support				
0-1	665 (27.2)	31.5	47.9	20.6
2	659 (26.7)	39.6	45.6	14.7
3-4	1167 (46.1)	50.9	36.8	12.2

Associations with skipping breakfast

In adjusted multinomial logistic regression analysis, being male was negatively associated with sometimes or mostly having breakfast. Experiencing hunger sometimes, soft drink consumption, short sleep and lack of parental support were associated with both sometimes or mostly and never or rarely having breakfast. Inadequate fruit and vegetable intake and physical inactivity were associated with sometimes or mostly having breakfast, and bullying victimization was associated with never or rarely having breakfast (see Table 2).

Table 2. Associations with skipping breakfast (versus daily breakfast)

Variable	Breakfast sometimes or mostly	Breakfast never or rarely	Breakfast sometimes or mostly	Breakfast never or rarely
	URRR (95% CI)	URRR (95% CI)	ARRR (95% CI)	ARRR (95% CI)
Sociodemographics				
Sex				
Female	1 (Reference)	1 (Reference)	1 (Reference)	1 (Reference)
Male	0.80 (0.66, 0.96)*	0.94 (0.74, 1.20)	0.79 (0.64, 0.97)*	1.00 (0.73, 1.37)
Age (years)				
≤14	1 (Reference)	1 (Reference)	1 (Reference)	1 (Reference)
15 or 16	1.24 (0.99, 1.56)	1.41 (1.10, 1.81)**	1.16 (0.87, 1.55)	1.16 (0.86, 1.58)
≥17	1.44 (1.12, 1.85)**	1.31 (0.99, 1.73)	1.29 (0.98, 1.69)	0.96 (0.64, 1.42)
Not live with both parents	1.23 1.01, 1.50)*	1.30 (1.01, 1.66)*	1.05 (0.85, 1.31)	1.17 (0.87, 1.59)
Parents provide necessities	0.68 (0.53, 0.88)**	0.50 (0.35, 0.73)***	0.75 (0.55, 1.02)	0.78 (0.50, 1.23)
Body weight and health risk behaviour				
Hungry				
Never or rarely	1 (Reference)	1 (Reference)	1 (Reference)	1 (Reference)
Sometimes	2.25 (1.68, 3.01)***	4.09 (2.93, 5.70)***	2.10 (1.39, 3.18)***	3.77 (3.49, 5.69)***
Mostly or always	1.75 (1.19, 2.56)**	2.76 (1.52, 5.01)***	1.22 (0.69, 2.17)	1.84 (0.94, 3.63)
Perceived body weight				
Normal	1 (Reference)	1 (Reference)	1 (Reference)	1 (Reference)
Underweight	1.05 (0.85, 1.29)	1.54 (1.06, 2.26)*	0.91 (0.69, 1.21)	1.28 (0.86, 1.91)
Overweight	1.07 (0.88, 1.31)	1.14 (0.88, 1.48)	0.92 (0.72, 1.18)	1.02 (0.76, 1.38)
Inadequate fruit and vegetable consumption	1.43 (1.09, 1.87)*	1.26 (0.88, 1.80)	1.41 (1.03, 1.92)*	1.43 (0.85, 2.39)
Trying to lose weight	0.91 (0.73, 1.13)	1.00 (0.75, 1.34)	---	---
Fast food consumption	1.20 (1.00, 1.45)	0.90 (0.74, 1.09)	---	---
Soft drink consumption	1.38 (1.08, 1.77)*	1.36 (1.07, 1.72)*	1.42 (1.12, 1.80)**	1.38 (1.02, 1.85)*

Table 2. (Continued)

Variable	Breakfast sometimes or mostly	Breakfast never or rarely	Breakfast sometimes or mostly	Breakfast never or rarely
	URRR (95% CI)	URRR (95% CI)	ARRR (95% CI)	ARRR (95% CI)
Current tobacco use	1.27 (0.97, 1.65)	1.54 (1.07, 2.21)*	0.91 (0.64, 1.31)	1.17 (0.66, 2.08)
Heavy alcohol use	1.05 (0.83, 1.34)	1.15 (0.79, 1.67)	---	---
Current cannabis use	1.31 (0.87, 1.98)	1.88 (1.17, 3.02)**	0.94 (0.53, 1.68)	1.11 (0.49, 2.57)
Sedentary behaviour	1.19 (0.98, 1.45)	1.10 (0.87, 1.40)	---	---
Physical inactivity	1.43 (1.13, 1.81)**	1.50 (1.04, 2.16)*	1.35 (1.04, 1.75)*	1.32 (0.87, 2.00)
Sleep duration				
Normal	1 (Reference)	1 (Reference)	1 (Reference)	1 (Reference)
Short	1.34 (1.11, 1.62)**	1.26 (1.00, 1.59)*	1.27 (1.00, 1.61)*	1.40 (1.03, 1.89)*
Very short	1.71 (1.30, 2.25)***	2.28 (1.64, 3.16)***	1.18 (0.83, 1.69)	1.87 (1.35, 2.60)***
Was bullied	1.25 (0.99, 1.59)	1.60 (1.27, 2.03)***	1.26 (0.97, 1.63)	1.39 (1.02, 1.89)*
Protective factors				
School attendance	0.71 (0.57, 0.90)**	0.63 (0.47, 0.85)**	0.85 (0.65, 1.10)	0.81 (0.55, 1.18)
Peer support	0.86 (0.74, 1.01)	0.57 (0.45, 0.71)***	1.07 (0.88, 1.29)	0.77 (0.59, 1.02)
Religious person	0.78 (0.65, 0.94)**	0.63 (0.49, 0.82)***	0.85 (0.68, 1.07)	0.75 (0.54, 1.02)
Parental support				
0-1	1 (Reference)	1 (Reference)	1 (Reference)	1 (Reference)
2	0.76 (0.57, 0.99)*	0.57 (0.42, 0.76)***	0.80 (0.59, 1.10)	0.75 (0.51, 1.10)
3-4	0.47 (0.38, 0.60)***	0.37 (0.27, 0.49)***	0.51 (0.38, 0.68)***	0.55 (0.41, 0.76)***

URRR=Unadjusted relative risk ratio; ARRR=Adjusted relative risk ratio; CI=Confidence Interval; ***P<0.001, **P<0.01, *P<0.05.

DISCUSSION

The study found a high prevalence of skipping breakfast (56.9%) in this nationally representative sample of in-school adolescents in Curaçao, which seem to be higher than in previous studies among adolescents in 39 European states (45%) (7), Finland (31.6% in girls and 16.5% in boys) (8), Jordan (34.3%) (9), in low- and middle-income countries (among girls 40.3%) (10), and among university students in three Caribbean countries (48.2% of females and 41.6% of males) (11). Some of these differences may be related to different definitions of breakfast skipping and different age groups.

In partial agreement with previous studies (8, 13-15), this study found that female sex and in unadjusted analysis older age were associated with skipping breakfast. It is possible that girls are more weight and/or body image conscious and engage therefore more likely than boys in skipping breakfast (13). To confirm this, however, we would have expected a positive relationship between dieting or trying to lose weight and skipping breakfast in this study, but no association was found. Considering the experience of hunger as a proxy for low economic status, this study found in line with previous investigations (8, 13, 14), that low family socioeconomic status was associated with skipping breakfast. Several studies (13, 14) found an association between living in single-parent families and skipping breakfast, while in this study, this was only found in unadjusted analysis.

Contrary to some previous findings (8, 14-16), this investigation did not find an association between perceived underweight or overweight and skipping breakfast. It is possible that no significant results were found in this study because body weight was measured by self-perception and not measured. Consistent with previous investigations (13, 16), results of this study showed an association between inadequate fruit and vegetable intake, soft drink consumption and skipping breakfast. Unlike some previous studies (13, 16, 17), this study did not find an association between fast food consumption, trying to lose weight or dieting and skipping breakfast. While some previous studies (8, 13, 17) found an association between smoking, heavy alcohol use and skipping breakfast, this investigation did not find such an association.

In agreement with former studies (8, 13-18), this study found an association between physical inactivity, short sleep, being bullied and skipping breakfast. In terms of protective factors, high parental support was protective from skipping breakfast. Parental support should be included as one of the strategies to improve breakfast eating. In several ways, this study seems to confirm that skipping breakfast appears in a cluster with other unhealthy behaviours, such as soft drink consumption, inadequate fruit and vegetable intake, physical inactivity, and short sleep (13, 17).

Study limitations

The investigation was limited because of its cross-sectional design, the inclusion of only school-going adolescents and the self-reported assessments, including perceived body weight.

The study lacked of assessing the context and content of breakfast consumption, which will be important to include in future investigations.

CONCLUSION

Almost two in three students skipped breakfast, and several risk factors, such as being female, experiencing hunger sometimes, soft drink consumption, inadequate fruit and vegetable intake, physical inactivity, short sleep, bullied and lack of parental support, were identified that can be targeted in programmes to increase daily breakfast consumption. Provision of breakfast in schools may be an important component of school health promotion.

APPENDIX 1. VARIABLE DESCRIPTION

Variables	Question	Response options
	Outcome variable	
Skipping breakfast	"During the past 30 days, how often did you eat breakfast?"	"Never, rarely, sometimes, most of the time, always"
	Sociodemographic factors	
Age	"How old are you?"	"11 years old or younger to 18 years old or older"
Sex	"What is your sex?"	"Male, Female"
Not live with both parents	"Which adult family members do you live with?"	1=both my mother and father to 5=I do not live with any adult family members (coded 2-5=1 and 1=0)
Parents provide necessities	"During the past 30 days, how often did your parents or guardians provide for your necessities?"	"1= never to 5= always (coded 1–3=0 and 4–5=1)"
	Body weight and health risk behaviour	
Hunger	"During the past 30 days, how often did you go hungry because there was not enough food in your home?"	"1= never to 5= always (coded 1-2=1,3=2 and 4–5=3)"
Perceived body weight	"How do you describe your weight?"	1=very underweight to 5=very overweight) (coded 1-2=underweight, 3=normal, 4-5 overweight)
Fruits	"During the past 30 days, how many times per day did you usually eat fruit such as papaya, melon, banana, apples, grape, or pineapple?"	"1=I did not eat fruit during the past 30 days to 7=5 or more times per day"
Vegetables	"During the past 30 days, how many times per day did you usually eat vegetables, such as carrots, beans, tomato, cabbage, or pumpkin?"	"I did not eat vegetables during the past 30 days to 7=5 or more times per day"
Trying to lose weight	"Which of the following are you trying to do about your weight?"	"I am not trying to do anything about my weight, lose weight, gain weight, stay the same"
Fast food consumption	"During the past 7 days, on how many days did you eat food from a fast food restaurant, such as McDonalds, KFC, Burger King, Pizza Hut, or Wendy's?"	"0=0 days to 7=7 days (coded 0=0 and 1-7=1)"

Appendix 1. (Continued)

Variables	Question	Response options
	Body weight and health risk behaviour	
Soft drink consumption	"During the past 30 days, how many times per day did you usually drink carbonated soft drinks, such as Coke, Sprite, fria, monster, busta, RedBull, coco rico, and malta? (Do not include diet soft drinks.)"	1=I did not drink carbonated soft drinks during the past 30 days to 7=5 or more times per day (coded 1=once or more/day)
Current tobacco use	"During the past 30 days, on how many days did you smoke cigarettes/use any tobacco products other than cigarettes, such as cigars, cigarillos, or electronic cigarettes?"	"1=0 days to 7=All 30 days (coded 1=0 and 2-7=1)"
Heavy alcohol use (2 or more/day)	"During the past 30 days, on the days you drink alcohol, how many drinks did you usually drink per day?"	1 = Not drink in the past 30 days to 7 = 5 or more drinks (coded 1–3 = 0 and 4–7 = 1)
Current cannabis use	"During the past 30 days, how many times have you used marijuana (also called weed, pot, cannabis, ganja, or grass)?"	"1=0 days to 7=All 30 days (coded 1=0 and 2-7=1)"
Leisure-time sedentary behaviour	"How much time do you spend during a typical or usual day sitting and watching television, playing computer games, talking with friends, or doing other sitting activities, such as playing domino?"	"1=Less than 1 hour per day… 3= 3 to 4 hours per day …6=8 or more hours a day"
Physical inactivity	"Physical activity is any activity that increases your heart rate and makes you get out of breath some of the time. Physical activity can be done in sports, playing with friends, or walking to school. Some examples of physical activity are running, fast walking, biking, dancing, football, swimming, baseball, and cross-fit. During the past 7 days, on how many days were you physically active for a total of at least 60 minutes per day?"	"0=0 days to 7=7 days (coded 0-6=1 and 7=0)"
Sleep duration	"On an average school night, how many hours of sleep do you get?"	"1=4 or less hours to 7=10 or more hours)"
Was bullied	"During the past 30 days, on how many days were you bullied?"	1=0 days to 7=All 30 days (coded 1=0 and 2–7=1)
	Protective factors	
School attendance	"During the past 30 days, on how many days did you miss classes or school without permission?"	"1=0 days to 5= 10 or more days (coded 1=1 and 2–5=0)"

Variables	Question	Response options
Protective factors		
Peer support	"During the past 30 days, how often were most of the students in your school kind and helpful?"	"1=never to 5=always (coded 1–3=0 and 4–5=1)"
Religious or spiritual person	"Do you think of yourself as a religious or spiritual person?"	"Yes, No"
Parental supervision	"During the past 30 days, how often did your parents or guardians check to see if your homework was done?"	"1=never to 5=always (coded 1–3=0 and 4–5=1)"
Parental connectedness	"During the past 30 days, how often did your parents or guardians understand your problems and worries?"	"1=never to 5=always (coded 1–3=0 and 4–5=1)"
Parental bonding	"During the past 30 days, how often did your parents or guardians really know what you were doing with your free time?	"1=never to 5=always (coded 1–3=0 and 4–5=1)"
Parental respect for privacy	"During the past 30 days, how often did your parents or guardians go through your things without your approval?"	"1=never to 5=always (coded 1–3=0 and 4–5=1)"

REFERENCES

[1] Gibney MJ, Barr SI, Bellisle F, Drewnowski A, Fagt S, Livingstone B, et al. Breakfast in human nutrition: The International Breakfast Research Initiative. Nutrients 2018;10(5). pii: E559. doi: 10.3390/nu10050559.

[2] Cayres SU, Júnior IF, Barbosa MF, Christofaro DG, Fernandes RA. Breakfast frequency, adiposity, and cardiovascular risk factors as markers in adolescents. Cardiol Young 2016;26(2):244-9. doi: 10.1017/S1047951115000050.

[3] Ballon A, Neuenschwander M, Schlesinger S. Breakfast skipping is associated with increased risk of type 2 diabetes among adults: A systematic review and meta-analysis of prospective cohort studies. J Nutr 2019;149(1):106-13. doi: 10.1093/jn/nxy194.

[4] Nurul-Fadhilah A, Teo PS, Huybrechts I, Foo LH. Infrequent breakfast consumption is associated is associated with higher adiposity and abdominal obesity in Malaysian school-aged adolescents. PLoS One 2013;8(3):e59297. doi: 10.1371/journal.pone.0059297.

[5] Takagi H, Hari Y, Nakashima K, Kuno T, Ando T; ALICE (All-Literature Investigation of Cardiovascular Evidence) Group. Meta-analysis of relation of skipping breakfast with heart disease. Am J Cardiol 2019;124(6):978-86. doi: 10.1016/j.amjcard.2019.06.016.

[6] Monzani A, Ricotti R, Caputo M, Solito A, Archero F, Bellone S, et al. A systematic review of the association of skipping breakfast with weight and cardiometabolic risk factors in children and adolescents. What should we better investigate in the future? Nutrients 2019;11(2). pii: E387. doi: 10.3390/nu11020387.

[7] Currie C, Zanotti C, Morgan A, Currie D, de Looze M, Roberts C, et al. Social determinants of health and well-being among young people. Copenhagen: WHO Regional Office Europe, 2012.

[8] Keski-Rahkonen A, Kaprio J, Rissanen A, Virkkunen M, Rose RJ. Breakfast skipping and health-compromising behaviors in adolescents and adults. Eur J Clin Nutr 2003;57(7):842-53.

[9] Ali RA, Abdel Razeq NM, Al-Kloub MI, Alzoubi FA. Predictors of breakfast skipping among 14 to 16 years old adolescents in Jordan: The influential role of mothers. Int J Nurs Pract 2019 Sep 12. doi: 10.1111/ijn.12778.

[10] Keats EC, Rappaport AI, Shah S, Oh C, Jain R, Bhutta ZA. The dietary intake and practices of adolescent girls in low- and middle-income countries: A systematic review. Nutrients 2018;10(12). pii: E1978. doi: 10.3390/nu10121978.

[11] Wright M, Adair L, James C, Amuleru-Marshall O, Peltzer K, Pengpid S, Samuels TA.The association of nutrition behaviors and physical activity with general and central obesity in Caribbean undergraduate students. Rev Panam Salud Publica 2015;38(4):278-85.

[12] Oba S, Oogushi K, Ogata H, Nakai H. Factors associated with irregular breakfast consumption among high school students in a Japanese community. Asia Pac J Clin Nutr 2016;25(1):165-73. doi: 10.6133/apjcn.2016.25.1.05.

[13] Vereecken C, Dupuy M, Rasmussen M, Kelly C, Nansel TR, Al Sabbah H, et al. Breakfast consumption and its socio-demographic and lifestyle correlates in schoolchildren in 41 countries participating in the HBSC study. Int J Public Health 2009;54(Suppl 2):180-90. doi: 10.1007/s00038-009-5409-5.

[14] Smith KJ, Breslin MC, McNaughton SA, Gall SL, Blizzard L, Venn AJ. Skipping breakfast among Australian children and adolescents; findings from the 2011-12 National Nutrition and Physical Activity Survey. Aust NZ J Public Health 2017;41(6):572-8. doi: 10.1111/1753-6405.12715.

[15] Tambalis KD, Panagiotakos DB, Psarra G, Sidossis LS. Breakfast skipping in Greek schoolchildren connected to an unhealthy lifestyle profile. Results from the National Action for Children's Health program. Nutr Diet 2019;76(3):328-35. doi: 10.1111/1747-0080.12522.

[16] Tin SP, Ho SY, Mak KH, Wan KL, Lam TH. Lifestyle and socioeconomic correlates of breakfast skipping in Hong Kong primary 4 schoolchildren. Prev Med 2011;52(3-4):250-3. doi: 10.1016/j.ypmed.2010.12.012.

[17] Kapantais E, Chala E, Kaklamanou D, Lanaras L, Kaklamanou M, Tzotzas T. Breakfast skipping and its relation to BMI and health-compromising behaviours among Greek adolescents. Public Health Nutr 2011;14(1):101-8. doi: 10.1017/S1368980010000765.

[18] Sampasa-Kanyinga H, Roumeliotis P, Farrow CV, Shi YF. Breakfast skipping is associated with cyberbullying and school bullying victimization. A school-based cross-sectional study. Appetite 2014;79:76-82. doi: 10.1016/j.appet.2014.04.007.

[19] World Health Organization (WHO). Global School-based Student Health Survey (GSHS). URL: http://www.who.int/chp/gshs/en/.

[20] Verstraeten S. The Curaçao Global School-based Student Health Survey (GSHS). Willemstad: Volksgezondheid Instituut Curaçao, 2015.

[21] Pengpid S, Peltzer K. Prevalence and correlates of behavioral non-communicable diseases risk factors among adolescents in the Seychelles: Results of a national school survey in 2015. Int J Environ Res Public Health 2019;16(15). pii: E2651. doi: 10.3390/ijerph16152651.

[22] World Health Organization (WHO) Diet, nutrition and the prevention of chronic diseases. Geneva, Switzerland: WHO, 2003.

[23] World Health Organization. Physical activity fact sheet, 2017. URL: http://www.who.int/mediacentre/factsheets/fs385/en/.

[24] Guthold R. Cowan MJ, Autenrieth CS, Kann L, Riley LM. Physical activity and sedentary behavior among schoolchildren: A 34-country comparison. J Pediatr 2010;157:43-9.

[25] National sleep foundation. National sleep foundation recommends new sleep times, 2019. URL: https://www.sleepfoundation.org/press-release/national-sleep-foundation-recommends-new-sleep-times/page/0/1.

In: Adolescence in Curaçao
Editors: Soraya Verstraeten et al.
ISBN: 978-1-53617-522-6

Chapter 13

SKIPPING BREAKFAST AND ITS ASSOCIATION WITH HEALTH RISK BEHAVIOUR AND MENTAL HEALTH AMONG SCHOOL-GOING ADOLESCENTS IN CURAÇAO: A CROSS-SECTIONAL NATIONAL STUDY

Karl Peltzer*[1]*, PhD and Supa Pengpid*[1,2,*]*, DrPH
[1]Department of Research Administration and Development, University of Limpopo, Turfloop, South Africa
[2]ASEAN Institute for Health Development, Mahidol University, Salaya, Phutthamonthon, Nakhon Pathom, Thailand

ABSTRACT

In this chapter we aim to investigate the associations between skipping breakfast and various health risk behaviours and mental health in

* ***Correspondence***: Professor Supa Pengpid, ASEAN Institute for Health Development, Mahidol University, 25/25 Phutthamonthon Road 4, Salaya, Phutthamonton, Nakhon Pathom 73170, Thailand. E-Mail: supaprom@yahoo.com.

adolescents in Curaçao. In the cross-sectional Curaçao "Global School-Based Student Health Survey (GSHS)" in 2015, 2,765 adolescents (median age 15 years) responded to questions on sociodemographic factors, mental health, health risk behaviours and protective factors. Results indicate that 56.9% of the students skipped breakfast (never, rarely, sometimes of most of the time had breakfast) in the past 30 days. In adjusted logistic regression analyses, skipping breakfast increased the odds for unhealthy dietary behaviours (inadequate fruit and vegetables intake, soft drink consumption, and fast food consumption), poor hand hygiene (not always washing hands before meals, after toilet and with soap), poor oral health hygiene (brushing teeth less <2 times/day, and not seeing a dentist in past year), not always wearing a seatbelt, and poor mental health indicators (anxiety, suicide ideation, suicide plan and short sleep). We found evidence that skipping breakfast was associated with ten of 15 health risk behaviours and four of six poor mental health indicators.

INTRODUCTION

In the adolescent period lifestyle patterns are developed, including breakfast consumption (1). Skipping breakfast is a common practice among adolescents, which has been shown in various studies, e.g., 45% in 39 European states (2) and 40.3% among adolescent girls in "low- and middle-income countries" (3), and significantly increases the risk of overweight/obesity, cardio metabolic risk factors, type 2 diabetes and heart disease (4-8). Few studies have investigated the association between skipping breakfast and health risk behaviour and mental health among adolescents in the Caribbean.

Various studies among adolescents found associations between skipping breakfast and overweight or obesity (5, 9-13), more negative body perception (11) and unhealthy dietary behaviour (14), including low fruit and vegetable intake (1, 11, 14, 15), higher sodium intake (14), lower consumption milk/dairy (1, 9, 14), higher consumption of sweets, sugary or soft drinks (1, 11), fast food consumption (1, 9), and skipping other meals (9, 11). Mental health correlates of skipping breakfast include stress or mentally distressed (16-18), depressive mood (13, 16, 19-21), suicidal ideation (16), suicide attempt (13), shorter sleep duration (1), and nocturnal sleeping problems (22).

Skipping breakfast has among adolescents further been associated with substance use, such as smoking (1, 10, 13) and alcohol use (1, 10, 13), physical inactivity (1, 9, 13, 23) and sedentary behaviour such as watch more television (9) and computer use (1). Other effects included poor oral hygiene, such as less frequent tooth brushing (24) and no dental care visit in the past year (25), and poor hand hygiene, such as no hand washing before meals (24), no seatbelt use (24), cardio metabolic risk factors, such as systolic blood pressure (4), and having low school grades (13, 17). The study aimed to investigate the associations between skipping breakfast and various health risk behaviours and mental health in adolescents in Curaçao.

OUR STUDY

Cross-sectional data from the 2015 Curaçao GSHS were analysed (26). The study used a two-stage cluster sampling approach to generate data that were representative of all students enrolled in public secondary education, comparable to US Grades 1-6, in Curaçao. "At the first stage, 28 schools were selected with probability proportional to enrolment size, and at the second stage, 161 classes were randomly selected" (27). All students in selected classes were eligible to participate after ethical approval in accordance with the *"WMA Declaration of Helsinki – Ethical Principles for Medical Research Involving Human Subjects"* and other permissions were granted and informed consent was obtained from parents and children; the overall response rate was 83% (27).

Measures

The GSHS measure was used in this survey (see Appendix 1) (26). "Inadequate FV consumption was classified as less than five or more servings in a day" (28, 29). "Inadequate physical activity was defined as not daily at least 60 minutes of moderate to vigorous-intensity physical activity."(30) "Sedentary behaviour was defined as spending three or more hours per day sitting."(31) Short sleep was defined as less than the normal or recommended sleep duration of "9-11 hours for 6-13 year-old children, 8-10 hours for 14-17 year-olds and 7-9 hours for 18-25 year-olds." (32) "The four items on parental or guardian support were summed, and classified into three groups, 0-1 low, 2 medium and 3-4 high support" (28).

Data analysis

Data analysis was conducted with "STATA software version 15.0 (Stata Corporation, College Station, TX, USA)," considering the complex study approach. Multivariable logistic regression was used to assess the associations between skipping breakfast categories (sometimes or mostly and never or rarely having breakfast), relevant confounders (age, sex, hunger, parental provision of necessities, living status, school attendance, being a religious or spiritual person, peer and parental support) and dependent variables (15 health risk behaviours and six poor mental health indicators). Missing data were excluded from the analysis. P values <0.05 were considered significant.

FINDINGS

The sample consisted of 2,765 school-going adolescents, 51.1% female and 48.9% male, 9.3% had sometimes and 3.8% had mostly or always experienced hunger in the past month, 81.7% had parents or guardians that provided them mostly or always with necessities, 49.9% lived with both parents, 69.0% considered themselves as religious or spiritual, 73.4% had always attended school I the past 30 days, 47.6% had peer support, 48.9% lived with both parents and 46.1% had high parental support. In all, 56.9% skipped breakfast (never, rarely, sometimes of most of the time had breakfast) in the past 30 days, 42.2% had sometimes or mostly breakfast and 14.9% had never or rarely had breakfast.

Table 1. Adjusted associations between skipping breakfast and health risk behaviours

Variable	AOR (95% CI)[1]	AOR (95% CI)[1]
	Breakfast sometimes or mostly	Breakfast never or rarely
Perceived body weight and health risk behaviour		
Inadequate fruit and vegetables intake (83.5%)	1.49 (1.11, 1.99)**	1.38 (0.94, 2.01)
Soft drink intake (≥1/day) (60.9%)	1.39 (1.10, 1.77)**	1.42 (1.10, 1.89)**
Fast food consumption (≥1/week) (69.0%)	1.33 (1.11, 1.60)**	0.91 (0.72, 1.15)
Perceived underweight (14.9%)	0.96 (0.75, 1.22)	1.23 (0.82, 1.83)
Perceived overweight (28.6%)	0.96 (0.77, 1.19)	0.98 (0.74, 1.29)
Heavy alcohol use (19.0%)	0.93 (0.74, 1.17)	0.95 (0.62, 1.45)
Current tobacco use (13.2%)	1.09 (0.82, 1.45)	1.17 (0.75, 1.80)
Not always wear seatbelt (71.9%)	1.42 (1.08, 1.88)*	1.46 (0.99, 2.16)
Not always washing hands before eating (68.7%)	1.40 (1.10, 1.79)**	1.54 (1.16, 2.06)**
Not always washing hands after toilet (33.3%)	1.20 (1.00, 1.44)*	1.32 (1.00, 1.75)*
Not always washing hands with soap (49.9%)	1.32 (1.08, 1.61)**	1.25 (0.97, 1.62)
Inadequate physical activity (88.2%)	1.34 (1.05, 1.71)*	1.37 (0.90, 2.08)
Sedentary behaviour (61.9%)	1.13 (0.89, 1.44)	1.02 (0.78, 1.32)
Tooth brushing <2 times/day (26.1%)	1.55 (1.23, 1.96)***	1.61 (1.17, 2.21)**
Saw dentist in the past 12 months (47.4%)	0.85 (0.69, 1.04)	0.68 (0.51, 0.90)**
Mental health		
Anxiety (11.4%)	1.59 (1.15, 2.18)**	1.81 (1.18, 2.79)**
Loneliness (15.5%)	1.06 (0.81, 1.38)	1.35 (0.93, 1.96)
Suicide ideation (11.3%)	1.00 (0.74, 1.34)	1.71 (1.17, 2.49)**
Suicide plan (9.1%)	1.19 (0.84, 1.68)	1.61 (1.02, 2.55)*
Suicide attempt (10.8%)	1.26 (0.88, 1.80)	1.34 (0.89, 2.01)
Short sleep (63.3%)	1.31 (1.05, 1.62)*	1.63 (1.25, 2.13)***

AOR=Adjusted Odds Ratio; ***P<0.001; **P<0.01; *P<0.05; [1]Adjusted for age, sex, hunger, parental provision of necessities, living status (not with both parents), religious person, school attendance, peer and parental support.

Associations between skipping breakfast and health risk behaviour and mental health

In adjusted logistic regression analyses, skipping breakfast (sometimes or mostly and/or never or rarely) increased the odds for unhealthy dietary behaviours (inadequate fruit and vegetables intake, soft drink consumption, and fast food consumption), poor hand hygiene (not always washing hands before meals, after toilet and with soap), poor oral healt hygiene (brushing teeth less <2 times/day, and not seeing a dentist in past year), and not always wearing a seatbelt.

Regarding mental health, skipping breakfast (sometimes or mostly and/or never or rarely) increased the odds for anxiety, suicide ideation, suicide plan and short sleep (see Table 1).

DISCUSSION

In agreement with a number of previous studies (1, 9, 11, 13-21, 23-25), this study found that skipping breakfast the likelihood of ten of 15 health risk behaviours and four of six poor mental health indicators. These findings replicate earlier results showing the wide range of possible effects of skipping breakfast on various health risk behaviours and poor mental indicators (14, 16, 18, 24).

Possible mechanisms to explain the effects of skipping breakfast on health risk behaviours and mental health, may be that having breakfast assists adolescents to "function better cognitively and psychosocially" (16, 33). This study suggests that skipping breakfast is part of an unhealthy behaviour pattern, including poor mental health, which clusters in the form of multiple risk behaviours (14, 24). However, various previous studies found an association between skipping breakfast and overweight or obesity (5, 9-13), and substance use (smoking and alcohol use) (1, 10, 13), while this study did not find any association.

Study limitations

The GSHS is limited to participants attending school, which does not include out-off school adolescents. The questionnaire administered was by self-report, and therefore some of the responses may have been biased. Skipping breakfast was only assessed with one question and did not include diet quality and information about other meals, and future studies should consider several questions, including diet quality, information about other meals, and provide definitions of terminology, such as what constitutes breakfast. The survey data were limited to cross-sectional design.

CONCLUSION

This investigation added evidence for an adolescent population in a Caribbean country that skipping breakfast was associated with ten of 15 health risk behaviours and four of six poor mental health indicators. Interventions programmes targeting breakfast consumption in adolescents should address linked health risk behaviours identified in Curaçao.

APPENDIX 1. VARIABLE DESCRIPTION

Variables	Question	Response options
Sociodemographic and protective factors		
Age	"How old are you?"	"11 years old or younger to 18 years old or older"
Sex	"What is your sex?"	"Male, Female"
Hunger	"During the past 30 days, how often did you go hungry because there was not enough food in your home?"	"1= never to 5= always (coded 1–3=0 and 4–5=1)"
Provision of necessities	"During the past 30 days, how often did your parents or guardians provide for your necessities?"	"1= never to 5= always (coded 1–3=0 and 4–5=1)"

Appendix 1. (Continued)

Variables	Question	Response options
Sociodemographic and protective factors		
Lives with both parents	"Which adult family members do you live with?"	1=both my mother and father to 5=I do not live with any adult family members (coded 2-5=0 and 1=1)
Religious or spiritual person	"Do you think of yourself as a religious or spiritual person?"	"Yes, No"
School attendance	"During the past 30 days, on how many days did you miss classes or school without permission?"	"1=0 days to 5= 10 or more days (coded 1=1 and 2–5=0)"
Peer support	"During the past 30 days, how often were most of the students in your school kind and helpful?"	"1=never to 5=always (coded 1–3=0 and 4–5=1)"
Parental supervision	"During the past 30 days, how often did your parents or guardians check to see if your homework was done?"	"1=never to 5=always (coded 1–3=0 and 4–5=1)"
Parental connectedness	"During the past 30 days, how often did your parents or guardians understand your problems and worries?"	"1=never to 5=always (coded 1–3=0 and 4–5=1)"
Parental bonding	"During the past 30 days, how often did your parents or guardians really know what you were doing with your free time?	"1=never to 5=always (coded 1–3=0 and 4–5=1)"
Parental respect for privacy	"During the past 30 days, how often did your parents or guardians go through your things without your approval?"	"1=never to 5=always (coded 1–3=0 and 4–5=1)"
Predictor variable		
Skipping breakfast	"During the past 30 days, how often did you eat breakfast?"	"Never, rarely, sometimes, most of the time, always"
Outcome variables		
Fruits	"During the past 30 days, how many times per day did you usually eat fruit such as papaya, melon, banana, apples, grape, or pineapple?"	"1=I did not eat fruit during the past 30 days to 7=5 or more times per day"
Vegetables	"During the past 30 days, how many times per day did you usually eat vegetables, such as carrots, beans, tomato, cabbage, or pumpkin?"	"I did not eat vegetables during the past 30 days to 7=5 or more times per day "
Soft drink consumption	"During the past 30 days, how many times per day did you usually drink carbonated soft drinks, such as Coke, Sprite, fria, monster, busta, RedBull, coco rico, and malta? (Do not include diet soft drinks.)"	1=I did not drink carbonated soft drinks during the past 30 days to 7=5 or more times per day (coded 1=once or more/day)

Variables	Question	Response options
	Outcome variables	
Fast food consumption	"During the past 7 days, on how many days did you eat food from a fast food restaurant, such as McDonalds, KFC, Burger King, Pizza Hut, or Wendy's?"	"0=0 days to 7=7 days (coded 0=0 and 1-7=1)"
Perceived body weight	"How do you describe your weight?"	1=very underweight to 5=very overweight) (coded 1-2=underweight, 3=normal, 4-5 overweight)
Heavy alcohol use (2 or more/day)	"During the past 30 days, on the days you drink alcohol, how many drinks did you usually drink per day?"	1 = Not drink in the past 30 days to 7 = 5 or more drinks (coded 1–3 = 0 and 4–7 = 1)
Current tobacco use	"During the past 30 days, on how many days did you smoke cigarettes/use any tobacco products other than cigarettes, such as cigars, cigarillos, or electronic cigarettes?"	"1=0 days to 7=All 30 days (coded 1=0 and 2-7=1)"
Not always wearing a seatbelt	"During the past 30 days, how often did you use a seat belt when riding in a car or other motor vehicle driven by someone else?"	1=Not apply, 2=never to 6=always (coded 2-5=1 and 1 and 6=0)
Hand washing before eating	"During the past 30 days, how often did you wash your hands before eating?"	"1=never to 5=always (coded 1–4=1 and 5=0)"
Hand washing after toilet	"During the past 30 days, how often did you wash your hands after using the toilet or latrine?"	"1=never to 5=always (coded 1–4=1 and 5=0)"
Using soap when hand washing	"During the past 30 days, how often did you use soap when washing your hands?"	"1=never to 5=always (coded 1–4=1 and 5=0)"
Physical inactivity	"Physical activity is any activity that increases your heart rate and makes you get out of breath some of the time. Physical activity can be done in sports, playing with friends, or walking to school. Some examples of physical activity are running, fast walking, biking, dancing, football, swimming, baseball, and cross-fit. During the past 7 days, on how many days were you physically active for a total of at least 60 minutes per day?"	"0=0 days to 7=7 days (coded 0-6=1 and 7=0)"
Leisure-time sedentary behavior	"How much time do you spend during a typical or usual day sitting and watching television, playing computer games, talking with friends, or doing other sitting activities, such as playing domino?"	"1=Less than 1 hour per day… 3= 3 to 4 hours per day …6=8 or more hours a day"
Tooth brushing (<2 times/day)	"During the past 30 days, how many times per day did you usually clean or brush your teeth?"	1=never to 6=4 or more times/day) (coded 1-3=1 and 4-6=0)

Appendix 1. (Continued)

Variables	Question	Response options
Outcome variables		
Saw dentist in the past 12 months	"When was the last time you saw a dentist for a check-up, exam, teeth cleaning, or other dental work?"	1=During the past 12 month to 4=never (coded 1=1 and 2-4=0)
Anxiety	"During the past 12 months, how often have you been so worried about something that you could not sleep at night?"	"1=never to 5=always (coded 1–3=0 and 4–5=1)"
Loneliness	"During the past 12 months, how often have you felt lonely?"	"1=never to 5=always (coded 1–3=0 and 4–5=1)"
Suicide ideation	"During the past 12 months, did you ever seriously consider attempting suicide?"	"Yes, No"
Suicide plan	"During the past 12 months, did you make a plan about how you would attempt suicide?"	"Yes, No"
Suicide attempt	"During the past 12 months, how many times did you actually attempt suicide?"	"1=0 times to 5=6 or more times (coded 1=0 and 2–5=1)"
Sleep duration	"On an average school night, how many hours of sleep do you get?"	"1=4 or less hours to 7=10 or more hours)"

REFERENCES

[1] Wang M, Zhong JM, Wang H, Zhao M, Gong WW, Pan J, et al. Breakfast consumption and its associations with health-related behaviors among school-aged adolescents: A cross-sectional study in Zhejiang Province, China. Int J Environ Res Public Health 2016;13(8). pii: E761. doi: 10.3390/ijerph13080761.

[2] Currie C, Zanotti C, Morgan A, Currie D, de Looze M, Roberts C, et al. Social determinants of health and well-being among young people. Copenhagen: WHO Regional Office for Europe; Copenhagen, 2012.

[3] Keats EC, Rappaport AI, Shah S, Oh C, Jain R, Bhutta ZA. The dietary intake and practices of adolescent girls in low- and middle-income countries: A systematic review. Nutrients 2018;10(12). pii: E1978. doi: 10.3390/nu10121978.

[4] Cayres SU, Júnior IF, Barbosa MF, Christofaro DG, Fernandes RA. Breakfast frequency, adiposity, and cardiovascular risk factors as markers in adolescents. Cardiol Young 2016;26(2):244-9. doi: 10.1017/S1047951115000050.

[5] Nurul-Fadhilah A, Teo PS, Huybrechts I, Foo LH. Infrequent breakfast consumption is associated with higher body adiposity and abdominal obesity in Malaysian school-aged adolescents. PLoS One 2013;8(3):e59297. doi: 10.1371/journal.pone.0059297.

[6] Ballon A, Neuenschwander M, Schlesinger S. Breakfast skipping is associated with increased risk of type 2 diabetes among adults: A systematic review and meta-analysis of prospective cohort studies. J Nutr 2019;149(1):106-13. doi: 10.1093/jn/nxy194.

[7] Monzani A, Ricotti R, Caputo M, Solito A, Archero F, Bellone S, et al. A systematic review of the association of skipping breakfast with weight and cardiometabolic risk factors in children and adolescents. What should we better investigate in the future? Nutrients 2019;11(2). pii: E387. doi: 10.3390/nu11020387.

[8] Takagi H, Hari Y, Nakashima K, Kuno T, Ando T; ALICE (All-Literature Investigation of Cardiovascular Evidence) Group. Meta-analysis of relation of skipping breakfast with heart disease. Am J Cardiol 2019;124(6):978-86. doi: 10.1016/j.amjcard.2019.06.016.

[9] Tin SP, Ho SY, Mak KH, Wan KL, Lam TH. Lifestyle and socioeconomic correlates of breakfast skipping in Hong Kong primary 4 schoolchildren. Prev Med 2011;52(3-4):250-3. doi: 10.1016/j.ypmed.2010.12.012.

[10] Kapantais E, Chala E, Kaklamanou D, Lanaras L, Kaklamanou M, Tzotzas T. Breakfast skipping and its relation to BMI and health-compromising behaviours among Greek adolescents. Public Health Nutr 2011;14(1):101-8. doi: 10.1017/S1368980010000765.

[11] van Vliet JS, Gustafsson PA, Nelson N. Feeling 'too fat' rather than being 'too fat' increases unhealthy eating habits among adolescents - even in boys. Food Nutr Res 2016;60:29530. doi: 10.3402/fnr.v60.29530. eCollection 2016.

[12] Yang RJ, Wang EK, Hsieh YS, Chen MY. Irregular breakfast eating and health status among adolescents in Taiwan. BMC Public Health 2006;6:295.

[13] Lee H J, Kim C H, Han I, Kim S H. Emotional state according to breakfast consumption in 62276 South Korean adolescents. Iran J Pediatr 2019;29(6):e92193. doi: 10.5812/ijp.92193.

[14] Rodrigues PRM, Luiz RR, Monteiro LS, Ferreira MG, Gonçalves-Silva RMV, Pereira RA. Adolescents' unhealthy eating habits are associated with meal skipping. Nutrition 2017;42:114-20.e1. doi: 10.1016/j.nut.2017.03.011.

[15] Pedersen TP, Meilstrup C, Holstein BE, Rasmussen M. Fruit and vegetable intake is associated with frequency of breakfast, lunch and evening meal: cross-sectional study of 11-, 13-, and 15-year-olds. Int J Behav Nutr Phys Act 2012;9:9. doi: 10.1186/1479-5868-9-9.

[16] Lee G, Han K, Kim H. Risk of mental health problems in adolescents skipping meals: The Korean National Health and Nutrition Examination Survey 2010 to 2012. Nurs Outlook 2017;65(4):411-9. doi: 10.1016/j.outlook.2017.01.007.

[17] Lien L. Is breakfast consumption related to mental distress and academic performance in adolescents? Public Health Nutr 2007;10(4):422-8.

[18] Tajik E, Latiffah AL, Awang H, Siti Nur'Asyura A, Chin YS, Azrin Shah AB, et al. Unhealthy diet practice and symptoms of stress and depression among adolescents in

Pasir Gudang, Malaysia. Obes Res Clin Pract 2016;10(2):114-23. doi: 10.1016/j.orcp.2015.06.001.

[19] Perveen A, Hamzah HB, Ramlee F, Morgul E, Govindasamy P. Skipping breakfast and lack of physical activity; contributing factors of depressive symptoms among university students. Inter J Aca Res Business Soc Sci 2018;8(8):12–23.

[20] Khan A, Ahmed R, Burton NW. Prevalence and correlates of depressive symptoms in secondary school children in Dhaka City, Bangladesh. Ethn Health 2020;25(1):34-46. doi: 10.1080/13557858.2017.1398313.

[21] Zhu Z, Cui Y, Gong Q, Huang C, Guo F, Li W, et al. Frequency of breakfast consumption is inversely associated with the risk of depressive symptoms among Chinese university students: A cross-sectional study. PLoS One 2019;14(8): e0222014. https://doi.org/10.1371/journal.pone.0222014.

[22] Peltzer K, Pengpid S. Nocturnal sleep problems among university students from 26 countries. Sleep Breath 2015;19(2):499-508. doi: 10.1007/s11325-014-1036-3.

[23] Pengpid S, Peltzer K, Kassean HK, Tsala Tsala JP, Sychareun V, Müller-Riemenschneider F. Physical inactivity and associated factors among university students in 23 low-, middle- and high-income countries. Int J Public Health 2015;60(5):539-49. doi: 10.1007/s00038-015-0680-0.

[24] Jordão LMR, Malta DC, Freire MDCM. Clustering patterns of oral and general health-risk behaviours in Brazilian adolescents: Findings from a national survey. Community Dent Oral Epidemiol 2018;46(2):194-202. doi: 10.1111/cdoe.12354.

[25] Peltzer K, Pengpid S. Oral health behaviour and social and health factors in university students from 26 low, middle and high income countries. Int J Environ Res Public Health 2014;11(12):12247-60. doi: 10.3390/ijerph111212247.

[26] World Health Organization (WHO). Global School-based Student Health Survey (GSHS). URL: http://www.who.int/chp/gshs/en/.

[27] Verstraeten S. The Curaçao Global School-based Student Health Survey (GSHS). Willemstad: Volksgezondheid Instituut Curaçao, 2015.

[28] Pengpid S, Peltzer K. Prevalence and correlates of behavioral non-communicable diseases risk factors among adolescents in the Seychelles: Results of a national school survey in 2015. Int J Environ Res Public Health 2019;16(15). pii: E2651. doi: 10.3390/ijerph16152651.

[29] World Health Organization (WHO) Diet, nutrition and the prevention of chronic diseases. Geneva, Switzerland: WHO, 2003.

[30] World Health Organization. Physical activity fact sheet, 2017. URL: http://www.who.int/mediacentre/factsheets/fs385/en/.

[31] Guthold R. Cowan MJ, Autenrieth CS, Kann L, Riley LM. Physical activity and sedentary behavior among schoolchildren: A 34-country comparison. J Pediatr 2010;157:43-49.

[32] National sleep foundation. National sleep foundation recommends new sleep times, 2019. URL: https://www.sleepfoundation.org/press-release/national-sleep-foundation-recommends-new-sleep-times/page/0/1.

OUR STUDY

Cross-sectional data from the 2015 Curaçao GSHS were analysed [9]. The study used a two-stage cluster sampling approach generating nationally representative data of all students enrolled in public secondary education, comparable to US Grades 1-6, in Curaçao. "At the first stage, 28 schools were selected with probability proportional to enrolment size, and at the second stage, 161 classes were randomly selected" [10]. All students in selected classes were eligible to participate after ethical approval in accordance with the "WMA Declaration of Helsinki - Ethical Principles for Medical Research Involving Human Subjects" and other permissions were granted and written informed consent was obtained from parents and children; the overall response rate was 83% [10].

Measures

The measure used was from the GSHS [11] and is described in detail in Appendix 1. Suicide attempt was assessed with the question, "During the past 12 months, how many times did you actually attempt suicide?" (number of times) The four items asking about parental support were combined and categorized into "0-1 low, 2 medium and 3-4 high support."

Data analysis

Statistical analyses were conducted with "STATA software version 15.0 (Stata Corporation, College Station, Texas, USA)," considering the complex study design in the analysis. Frequency statistics was used to describe the sample. Predictors of suicide attempt in the past year were calculated with logistic regression analysis. Missing data were not included in the analysis. A $P < 0.05$ level was considered significant.

FINDINGS

The study sample comprised of 2,765 school-going adolescents (median age 15 years, interquartile range 3), 51.1% female and 48.9% male, 3.8% had mostly or always experienced hunger in the past month, and 81.7% had parents or guardians that provided them mostly or always with necessities. More than two thirds (69.0%) of students perceived themselves to be a religious or spiritual person, 47.6% received mostly or always peer support in the past month and 46.1% scored high on parental support. The prevalence of various psychosocial and social-environmental factors are described in Table 1. Overall, the prevalence of suicide attempt (past year) was 10.8%, 12.6% among females and 8.5% among males, and the prevalence of suicide ideation (past year) was 11.3% and suicide plan 9.1% (see Table 2).

Associations with suicide attempt

In adjusted logistic regression analysis, female sex, non-parental provision of necessities, loneliness, anxiety, in a physical fight, physical violence from parents, history of forced sexual intercourse, carrying a weapon and perceived overweight were associated with suicide attempt in the past year (see Table 3).

DISCUSSION

The study found a national prevalence of suicide attempt (past year) of 10.8% in Curaçao, which seems lower than in other school-based surveys among adolescents in Caribbean countries, ranging from 12.3% in Antigua and Barbuda to 24.1% in Jamaica [5]. Sociocultural differences between Caribbean countries may result in differences in the rate of suicide attempt, which should be investigated in future studies.

Table 1. Description of variables

Variables	Question	Response options (coding scheme)
Age	"How old are you?"	"11 years old or younger to 18 years old or older"
Sex	"What is your sex?"	"Male, Female"
Provision of necessities	"During the past 30 days, how often did your parents or guardians provide for your necessities?"	"1 = never to 5 = always (coded 1-3 = 0 and 4-5 = 1)"
Hunger	"During the past 30 days, how often did you go hungry because there was not enough food in your home?"	"1 = never to 5 = always (coded 1-3 = 0 and 4-5 = 1)"
Suicide ideation	"During the past 12 months, did you ever seriously consider attempting suicide?"	"Yes, No"
Suicide plan	"During the past 12 months, did you make a plan about how you would attempt suicide?"	"Yes, No"
Suicide attempt	"During the past 12 months, how many times did you actually attempt suicide?"	"1 = 0 times to 5 = 6 or more times (coded 1 = 0 and 2-5 = 1)"
Psychosocial distress		
No close friends	"How many close friends do you have?"	"1 = 0 to 4 = 3 or more (coded 1 + = 0, 0 = 1)"
Loneliness	"During the past 12 months, how often have you felt lonely?"	"1 = never to 5 = always (coded 1-3 = 0 and 4-5 = 1)"
Anxiety	"During the past 12 months, how often have you been so worried about something that you could not sleep at night?"	"1=never to 5=always (coded 1-3 = 0 and 4–5 = 1)"
Was bullied	"During the past 30 days, on how many days were you bullied?"	"1 = 0 days to 7 = All 30 days (coded 1 = 0 and 2-7 = 1)"
Was physically attacked	"During the past 12 months, how many times were you physically attacked?"	"1 = 0 times to 8 = 12 or more times (coded 1 = 0 and 2-8 = 1)"
Was in a physical fight	"During the past 12 months, how many times were you in a physical fight?"	"1 = 0 times to 8 = 12 or more times (coded 1 = 0 and 2-8 = 1)"
Physical violence from parents	"During the past 12 months, did your parents or guardians ever hit, slap, or physically hurt you on purpose?"	"Yes, No (coded yes = 1 and no = 0)"
Physical intimate partner violence victimization	"During the past 12 months, did your boyfriend or girlfriend ever hit, slap, or physically hurt you on purpose?"	"Yes, No"
Forced sexual intercourse	"Have you ever been forced to have sexual intercourse when you did not want to?"	"Yes, No" (coded yes = 1 and no = 0)"
Carried a weapon	"During the past 30 days, on how many days did you carry a weapon, such as a gun, knife, club, or brass knuckles?"	"1 = 0 days to 5 = 6 or more days"

Table 1. (Continued)

Variables	Question	Response options (coding scheme)
	Socio-environmental factors	
Parental supervision	"During the past 30 days, how often did your parents or guardians check to see if your homework was done?"	"1 = never to 5 = always (coded 1-3 = 0 and 4-5 = 1)"
Parental connectedness	"During the past 30 days, how often did your parents or guardians understand your problems and worries?"	"1 = never to 5 = always (coded 1-3 = 0 and 4-5 = 1)"
Parental bonding	"During the past 30 days, how often did your parents or guardians really know what you were doing with your free time?	"1 = never to 5 = always (coded 1-3 = 0 and 4-5 = 1)"
Parental respect for privacy	"During the past 30 days, how often did your parents or guardians go through your things without your approval?"	"1 = never to 5 = always (coded 1-3 = 0 and 4-5 = 1)"
Peer support	"During the past 30 days, how often were most of the students in your school kind and helpful?"	"1 = never to 5 = always (coded 1-3 = 0 and 4-5 = 1)"
Religious or spiritual person	"Do you think of yourself as a religious or spiritual person?"	"Yes, No"
Current tobacco use	"During the past 30 days, on how many days did you smoke cigarettes/use any tobacco products other than cigarettes, such as cigars, cigarillos, or electronic cigarettes?"	"1 = 0 days to 7 = All 30 days (coded 1 = 0 and 2-7 = 1)"
Heavy alcohol use (2 or more/day)	"During the past 30 days, on the days you drink alcohol, how many drinks did you usually drink per day?"	"1 = Not drink in the past 30 days to 7 = 5 or more drinks (coded 1-3 = 0 and 4-7 = 1)"
Current cannabis use	"During the past 30 days, how many times have you used marijuana?"	"1 = 0 times to 5 = 20 or more times (coded 1 = 0 and 2-5 = 1)"
Soft drinks	"During the past 30 days, how many times per day did you usually drink carbonated soft drinks, such as Coca-cola, Pepsi Cola, Sprite, Seven-up, Grapette, or Orange Crush? (Do not include diet soft drinks.)?"	"1 = not in the past days to 7 = 5 or more times per day (coded 1-3 = 0 and 4-7 = 1)"
Perceived body weight	"How do you describe your weight?"	"1 = very underweight to 5 = very overweight) (coded 1-2 = underweight, 3 = normal, 4-5 overweight)"
Truancy	"During the past 30 days, on how many days did you miss classes or school without permission?"	"1 = 0 days to 5 = 10 or more days (coded 1 = 0 and 2-5 = 1)"
Injury	"During the past 12 months, how many times were you seriously injured?" "(An injury is serious when it makes you miss at least one full day of usual activities (such as school, sports, or a job) or requires treatment by a doctor or nurse.)"	"1 = 0 times to 8 = 12 or more times (coded 1 = 0 and 2-8 = 1)"
Belong to violent group	"Do you belong to any violent group?"	"Yes, No"

Table 2. Sample and suicide attempt characteristics

Variables	Sample	Past 12-month suicide attempt
	N (%)	%
Socio-demographics		
All	2765	10.8
Sex		
Female	1508 (51.1)	12.6
Male	1230 (48.9)	8.5
Age in years		
≤11-14	1054 (32.8)	11.2
15-16	824 (32.7)	12.7
17-18 or more	877 (34.5)	8.3
Parents provide necessities	2082 (81.7)	8.7
Hunger	102 (3.8)	30.4
Psychosocial distress		
No close friends	265 (10.0)	16.4
Loneliness	417 (15.5)	26.0
Anxiety	306 (11.4)	27.3
Was bullied	683 (25.4)	19.1
Was physically attacked	394 (14.3)	23.0
Was in physical fight	492 (17.9)	19.3
Physical violence from parents	417 (15.2)	20.6
Physical intimate partner violence victimization	282 (10.5)	16.8
Forced sexual intercourse	159 (5.9)	27.7
Carried a weapon	363 (13.9)	22.9
Suicide ideation	308 (11.3)	51.1
Suicide plan	247 (9.1)	59.1
Social-environmental factors		
Parental/guardian support index		
0-1	665 (27.2)	15.7
2	659 (26.7)	10.3
3-4	1167 (46.1)	7.1
Peer support (mostly/always)	1241 (47.6)	8.4
Religious or spiritual person	1717 (69.0)	9.3
Current tobacco use	345 (13.2)	23.6
Heavy alcohol use	477 (19.0)	13.9
Current cannabis use	136 (5.7)	24.0
Soft drinks (1 or more/day)	1670 (60.9)	12.6
Perceived body weight		
Normal	1521 (56.5)	8.0
Underweight	400 (14.9)	16.1
Overweight	787 (28.6)	13.3
Truancy	652 (26.6)	15.0
Injury	808 (31.7)	16.8
Belongs to violent group	165 (6.1)	23.3

Table 3. Logistic regression for predictors of suicide attempts

Variables	COR (95% CI)	AOR (95% CI)[a]
Socio-demographics		
Sex		
Female	1 (Reference)	1 (Reference)
Male	0.64 (0.49, 0.84)**	0.51 (0.34, 0.77)**
Age in years		
≤11-14	1 (Reference)	---
15-16	1.16 (0.84, 1.61)	
17-18 or more	0.72 (0.49, 1.07)	
Parents provide necessities	0.43 (0.30, 0.62)***	0.62 (0.43, 0.90)*
Hunger	4.00 (2.51, 6.37)***	1.81 (0.80, 4.13)
Psychosocial distress		
No close friends	1.78 (1.24, 2.55)**	1.43 (0.84, 1.38)
Loneliness	4.15 (3.04, 5.67)***	2.43 (1.53, 3.86)***
Anxiety	4.04 (2.94, 5.54)***	1.62 (1.05, 2.50)*
Was bullied	2.93 (2.33, 3.69)***	1.20 (0.83, 1.73)
Was physically attacked	3.29 (2.40, 4.50)***	1.48 (0.88, 2.49)
Was in physical fight	2.45 (1.83, 3.28)***	1.60 (1.01, 2.45)*
Physical violence from parents	2.90 (2.19, 3.84)***	1.58 (1.08, 2.31)*
Physical intimate partner violence victimization	1.88 (1.31, 2.70)***	1.10 (0.66, 1.04)
Forced sexual intercourse	3.71 (2.48, 5.54)***	1.96 (1.06, 3.62)*
Carried a weapon	3.04 (2.21, 4.17)***	2.06 (1.35, 3.15)***
Social-environmental factors		
Parental/guardian support index		
0-1	1 (Reference)	1 (Reference)
2	0.62 (0.47, 0.81)***	0.92 (0.62, 1.38)
3-4	0.41 (0.29, 0.59)***	0.88 (0.52, 1.50)
Peer support (mostly/always)	0.68 (0.53, 0.87)**	1.03 (0.71, 1.48)
Religious or spiritual person	0.75 (0.55, 1.02)	---
Current tobacco use	3.21 (2.36, 4.36)***	1.74 (0.99, 3.05)
Heavy alcohol use	1.49 (1.07, 2.08)*	0.78 (0.45, 1.34)
Current cannabis use	2.92 (1.92, 4.43)***	0.99 (0.40, 2.44)
Soft drinks (1 or more/day)	1.70 (1.27, 2.27)***	1.39 (0.90, 2.16)
Perceived body weight		
Normal	1 (Reference)	1 (Reference)
Underweight	2.20 (1.48, 3.27)***	1.69 (0.93, 3.10)
Overweight	1.77 (1.22, 2.56)**	1.81 (1.11, 2.94)*
Truancy	1.80 (1.37, 2.36)***	0.78 (0.48, 1.26)
Injury	2.35 (1.77, 3.11)***	1.50 (0.96, 2.33)
Belongs to violent group	2.90 (2.04, 4.11)***	1.58 (0.63, 4.00)

COR: Crude Odds Ratio; AOR = Adjusted Odds Ratio; [a]Adjusted for all variables in the table; CI = Confidence Interval; *** $P < 0.001$; ** $P < 0.01$; * $P < 0.05$.

Most students with a suicide attempt had a suicide plan, which is consistent with previous findings [5, 8], and stresses the importance of early identification of suicide plans in suicide prevention efforts [5, 8]. In order to prevent suicide attempts of an impulsive nature, restricting access to suicide means will be relevant [5, 8]. This may, however, not be easy, since adolescents in Curaçao may have easy available pesticides as a means of attempting suicide; poisoning (47.3%) and suffocation (34.1%) being the two most common methods of suicide in the non-Hispanic Caribbean [12].

This investigation found a higher prevalence of suicide attempt in girls than in boys, which is consistent with previous studies [5, 13]. These sex differences may be related males being more likely to externalize psycho-behavioural problems (leading more likely to suicide death) and females more likely to internalize emotional-behavioural problems (leading more likely to suicidal ideation and suicide attempts) [14]. Consistent with previous results [5, 15], this study found that the parental provision of necessities was protective from suicide attempt. Further, in agreement with previous studies [5, 7, 13, 15-18], this study found an association between psychosocial distress (loneliness, anxiety and interpersonal violence, including was in physical fight, physical violence from parents, history of forced sexual intercourse and weapon carrying) and suicide attempt. These findings suggest the importance of treating psychosocial distress, the consequences of interpersonal violence, including rape, and precluding access to weapons in order to prevent suicide.

Unlike previous research [5, 16, 17, 19, 20], this study found did not find an association between substance use (alcohol, tobacco and cannabis), lack of parental or guardian support, lack of peer support and suicide attempts. A systematic review found that there is an "inverse association between obesity and overweight with attempted suicide and positive association between obesity and overweight with suicidal ideation" [21], while this study found a positive association between perceived overweight and suicide attempt. Some studies [6, 22] among adolescents in the Caribbean found that religious involvement (prayer with family, attendance of religious services) was protective from suicide attempt, this study did not find an association between being a religious or spiritual person and suicide attempt.

Study limitations

The study was limited to the cross sectional design and to public school-going youth. The study responses were assessed by self-report, including suicidal behaviour, psychosocial distress and social-environmental factors, which could have led to biased reporting. An additional limitation was that the GSHS in Curaçao did not assess help seeking behaviours for suicidal behaviours.

Conclusion

More than one in ten adolescents had attempted suicide in the past 12 month among in-school adolescents in Curaçao. Several risk factors for suicide attempt were identified, including being female, lack of parental provision of necessities, loneliness, anxiety, in physical fight, physical violence from parents, history of forced sexual intercourse, weapon carrying, and perceived overweight. These risk factors should be targeted in school health promotion programmes, in order to prevent attempting suicide in this adolescent population.

References

[1] World Health Organization (WHO). Adolescent mental health, 2019. URL: https://www.who.int/news-room/fact-sheets/detail/adolescent-mental-health.

[2] Bilsen J. Suicide and youth: Risk factors. *Front. Psychiatry* 2018;9: 540. doi: 10.3389/fpsyt.2018.00540. eCollection 2018.

[3] Hawton K, Saunders KE, O'Connor RC. Self-harm and suicide in adolescents. *Lancet* 2012;379(9834):2373-82.

[4] Mijangos MDF, Coguox LNC, Morales MRS, Patino DC, Torres AR. Suicide attempt: Sociodemographic/motivational description of case series in Santa Rosa, Guatemala. *Int. J. Curr. Adv. Res.* 2017; 6(4): 3474-7.

[5] Liu X, Huang Y, Liu Y. Prevalence, distribution, and associated factors of suicide attempts in young adolescents: School-based data from 40 low-income and middle-

income countries. *PLoS One* 2018; 13(12):e0207823. doi: 10.1371/journal.pone. 0207823. eCollection 2018.

[6] Ali A, Maharajh HD. Social predictors of suicidal behaviour in adolescents in Trinidad and Tobago. *Soc. Psychiatry Psychiatr. Epidemiol.* 2005;40(3):186-91.

[7] Kukoyi OY, Shuaib FM, Campbell-Forrester S, Crossman L, Jolly PE. Suicidal ideation and suicide attempt among adolescents in Western Jamaica: a preliminary study. *Crisis.* 2010;31(6):317-27. doi: 10.1027/0227-5910/a000038.

[8] Pengpid S, Peltzer K. Prevalence and correlates of past 12-month suicide attempt among in-school adolescents in Guatemala. *Psychol. Res. Behav. Manag.* 2019;12:523-9. doi: 10.2147/PRBM.S212648. eCollection 2019.

[9] World Health Organization (WHO) Global School-based Student Health Survey (GSHS). 2015 Curacao. URL: https://www.who.int/ ncds/surveillance/gshs/ curacaodataset/en/.

[10] Verstraeten S. National report the Curaçao Global School-based Student Health Survey (GSHS) study 2015. URL: https://www.who. int/ncds/surveillance/gshs/ Final_report_2015_GSHS_Curacao.pdf.

[11] World Health Organization (WHO) Global School-based Student Health Survey (GSHS). 2015 Curacao GSHS Questionnaire. URL: https://www.who.int/ncds/ surveillance/gshs/2015_GSHS_Curacao_Questionnaire.pdf.

[12] Pan American Health Organization. Suicide mortality in the Americas, 2014. URL: https://www.paho.org/hq/dmdocuments/2015/ suicide-PAHO-mortality-2014.pdf.

[13] Miranda-Mendizabal A, Castellví P, Parés-Badell O, Alayo I, Almenara J, Alonso I, et al. Gender differences in suicidal behavior in adolescents and young adults: systematic review and meta-analysis of longitudinal studies. *Int. J. Public Health* 2019;64(2):265-283. doi: 10.1007/s00038-018-1196-1.

[14] Kaess M, Parzer P, Haffner J Steen R, Roos J, Klett M, Brunner R, Resch F. Explaining gender differences in non-fatal suicidal behaviour among adolescents: a population-based study. *BMC Public Health* 2011;11:597. https://doi. org/10.1186/ 1471-2458-11-597.

[15] Oppong Asante K, Kugbey N Osafo J, Quarshie EN, Sarfo JO. The prevalence and correlates of suicidal behaviours (ideation, plan and attempt) among adolescents in senior high schools in Ghana. *SSM Population Health* 2017;3:427-34. doi: 10.1016/j.ssmph.2017.05. 005. eCollection 2017 Dec.

[16] Reyes JC, Robles RR, Colón HM, Negrón JL, Matos TD, Calderón JM. Polydrug use and attempted suicide among Hispanic adolescents in Puerto Rico. *Arch. Suicide Res.* 2011;15(2):151-9. doi: 10.1080/ 13811118.2011.565274.

[17] Randall JR, Doku D, Wilson ML, Peltzer K. Suicidal behaviour and related risk factors among school-aged youth in the Republic of Benin. *PLoS One* 2014;9(2): e88233.

[18] Sharma B, Nam EW, Kim HY, Kim JK. Factors associated with suicidal ideation and suicide attempt among school-going urban adolescents in Peru. *Int. J. Environ. Res. Public Health* 2015;12(11): 14842-56. doi: 10.3390/ijerph121114842.

[19] Carballo JJ, Llorente C, Kehrmann L, Flamarique I, Zuddas A, Purper-Ouakil D, et al. Psychosocial risk factors for suicidality in children and adolescents. *Eur. Child Adolesc. Psychiatry* 2019. doi: 10.1007/s00787-018-01270-9.

[20] Carvalho AF, Stubbs B, Vancampfort D, Kloiber S, Maes M, Firth J, et al. Cannabis use and suicide attempts among 86,254 adolescentsaged 12-15 years from 21 low- and middle-income countries. *Eur. Psychiatry* 2019;56:8-13. doi: 10.1016/j.eurpsy.2018. 10.006.

[21] Amiri S, Behnezhad S. Body mass index and risk of suicide: A systematic review and meta-analysis. *J. Affect. Disord.* 2018;238: 615-25. doi: 10.1016/j.jad. 2018.05.028.

[22] Toussaint L, Wilson CM, Wilson LC, Williams DR. Religiousness and suicide in a nationally representative sample of Trinidad and Tobago adolescents and young adults. *Soc. Psychiatry Psychiatr. Epidemiol.* 2015;50(9):1441-50. doi: 10.1007/s00127-015-1045-y.

In: Adolescence in Curaçao
Editors: Soraya Verstraeten et al.
ISBN: 978-1-53617-522-6

Chapter 15

UNINTENTIONAL INJURIES AND ASSOCIATED FACTORS AMONG IN-SCHOOL ADOLESCENTS IN CURAÇAO: A NATIONAL CROSS-SECTIONAL STUDY

Supa Pengpid*[1,2], *DrPH and Karl Peltzer*[*,2], *PhD

[1]ASEAN Institute for Health Development, Mahidol University, Salaya, Phutthamonthon, Nakhon Pathom, Thailand

[2]Department of Research Administration and Development, University of Limpopo, Turfloop, South Africa

ABSTRACT

In this chapter we aim to report on the prevalence and associated factors of non-fatal injury among in-school adolescents in Curaçao. In the cross-sectional Curaçao "Global School-Based Student Health Survey (GSHS)" in 2015, 2,765 adolescents (median age 15 years) responded to questions

---

* ***Correspondence***: Professor Karl Peltzer, Department of Research Administration and Development, University of Limpopo, Turfloop Campus, Private Bag X1106, Sovenga 0727, South Africa. Email: kfpeltzer@gmail.com.

on sociodemographic factors, frequency, cause and type of injury, substance use and other health risk behaviour, psychological distress, and protective factors. Results indicate that the prevalence of one or multiple injuries in the past year was 31.7%. The most frequent cause of the reported injury was fall (6.4%), followed by "struck or hit by object" (2.3%) and "traffic injury" (1.9%), and the most common types of injury were "fracture or dislocation" (4.5%), "cut or stab wound" (4.2%), and concussion (1.7%). In adjusted logistic regression analysis, younger age, male sex, heavy alcohol use, current cannabis use, adequate physical activity and psychological distress were associated with injury. Almost one in three of the participants had sustained at least one serious injury in the past 12 months and various factors were found that could be targeted in programmes addressing injury prevention.

INTRODUCTION

Unintentional injuries contribute to a large burden of death among adolescents (1). In a large study among school-going adolescents in 68 "low- and middle-income countries", the overall prevalence of serious injury (past year) was 42.9% (2). "Violence and injuries have become a huge burden on the state and society throughout the Caribbean" (3). Among in-school adolescents in seven Caribbean countries, the injury (past year) prevalence was 54.3%, ranging "from 43.1% in Dominica to 59.5% in Jamaica" (4). There are is a dearth of studies on the prevalence and correlates of unintentional injuries in Curaçao.

Factors associated with unintentional injury in adolescents may include, "sociodemographic variables, such as male sex and lower economic status and socio-psychological factors such as psychological distress, alcohol and tobacco use, and risk-taking behaviours."(5) In the seven country study among adolescents in the Caribbean, the leading external causes of injury included "fall" (11.4%), fighting (5.0%), "something fell on me or hit me"(4.9%) and traffic accident (4.3%), and the three most common types of injuries were a "cut, puncture, stab wound" (9.5%), "broken bone/dislocated joint" (7.8%) and "concussion/head injury" (2.7%) (4). The study aimed to report on the prevalence and associated factors of non-fatal injury among in-school adolescents in Curaçao.

Our study

Cross-sectional data from the 2015 Curaçao GSHS were analysed (6). The study used a two-stage cluster sampling approach to generate representative data of all students enrolled in public secondary education, comparable to US Grades 1-6, in Curaçao. "At the first stage, 28 schools were selected with probability proportional to enrolment size, and at the second stage, 161 classes were randomly selected" (7). All students in the selected school classes were eligible to participate after ethical approval in accordance with the *"WMA Declaration of Helsinki – Ethical Principles for Medical Research Involving Human Subjects"* and other permissions were granted and informed consent was obtained from parents and children; the overall response rate was 83% (7).

Measures

The GSHS measure was used in this survey (Appendix 1) (8). "Adequate physical activity was defined as daily at least 60 minutes of moderate to vigorous-intensity physical activity."(9) "The psychological distress items (no close friends, loneliness, anxiety, suicidal ideation and suicide attempt) were summed, and grouped into 0 = 0, 1 = 1 single and 2-5 = 2 multiple."(10) "The four items on parental or guardian support were summed, and classified into three groups, 0-1 low, 2 medium and 3-4 high support." (10) The experience of hunger and provision of necessities assessed were used as a proxy for socioeconomic status.

Data analysis

Data analysis was conducted using "STATA software version 15.0 (Stata Corporation, College Station, Texas, USA)", considering the complex sampling strategy. Frequency distributions are used to describe the sample. Logistic regression was utilized to calculate associations between independent variables and dependent variable (≥ 1 injuries/past year). Independent variables found significant in bivariate analysis were subsequently incorporated in the final regression model. $P < 0.05$ was considered significant.

FINDINGS

The study sample comprised of 2,765 school-going adolescents, with a median age of 15 years (interquartile range = 3), 51.1% female and 48.9% male, 3.8% had (mostly or always) experienced hunger (past month), and 81.7% had parents or guardians that provided them mostly or always with necessities. The prevalence of having sustained one or multiple injuries in the past year was 31.7%. The most frequent cause of the reported injury was fall (6.4%), followed by "struck or hit by object" (2.3%) and "traffic injury" (1.9%). The prevalence of fall and "struck or hit by object" was significantly higher in boys than girls. The most prevalent type of injury was "fracture or dislocation" (4.5%), followed by "cut or stab wound" (4.2%), and concussion (1.7%). The prevalence of "fracture or dislocation" and "cut or stab wound" was significantly higher in boys than girls (see table 1).

Associations with one or multiple injuries

In adjusted logistic regression analysis, younger age, male sex, heavy alcohol use, current cannabis use, adequate physical activity and psychological distress increased the odds for injury (see table 2).

Table 1. Annual prevalence of injury events, cause and type of injury by sex, Curaçao, 2015

Variable	Total	Boys	Girls
	% (95% CI)	% (95% CI)	% (95% CI)
INJURY (in the past 12 months)			
Injured once or more times	31.7 (29.4, 34.1)	37.4 (40.9)	26.2 (24.3, 28.1)
CAUSE (of most serious injury)			
"Traffic injury"	1.9 (1.3, 2.8)	1.9 (1.2, 3.0)	2.0 (1.2, 3.2)
"Fall"	6.4 (5.3, 7.8)	9.0 (7.2, 11.2)	4.2 (3.0, 5.7)
"Struck/hit by object"	2.3 (1.7, 3.3)	3.7 (2.6, 5.4)	1.0 (0.7, 1.6)
"Struck/hit by person"	0.7 (0.4, 1.2)	1.1 (0.6, 2.0)	0.3 (0.1, 1.6)
"Fire, flames or heat"	0.5 (0.3, 0.8)	0.2 (0.04, 0.8)	0.7 (0.4, 1.3)
"Poisoning"	0.6 (0.3, 1.0)	0.5 (0.2, 1.0)	0.7 (0.3, 1.3)
"Other"	14.6 (13.1, 16.1)	15.4 (13.3, 17.8)	13.6 (11.9, 15.6)
TYPE OF INJURY (of most serious injury)			
"Fracture or dislocation"	4.5 (3.5, 5.7)	6.5 (5.0, 8.4)	2.5 (1.7, 3.8)
"Cut or stab wound"	4.2 (3.5, 5.0)	6.5 (5.2, 8.0)	2.1 (1.5, 3.0)
"Concussion"	1.7 (1.2, 2.3)	1.4 (0.9, 2.3)	1.7 (1.1, 2.6)
"Gunshot wound"	0.5 (0.4, 2.3)	0.7 (0.2, 2.0)	0.1 (0.04, 0.6)
"Burns"	0.6 (0.3, 1.1)	0.5 (0.1, 1.4)	0.6 (0.3, 1.2)
"Poisoned"	0.2 (0.1, 0.6)	0.3 (0.09, 1.0)	0.2 (0.07, 0.7)
"Other"	15.7 (14.2, 17.2)	16.5 (14.3, 19.0)	15.1 (13.3, 17.2)

CI = Confidence Interval.

DISCUSSION

The study reported for the first time the national prevalence of non-fatal injuries among in-school adolescents in Curaçao, showing a lower prevalence of injury (31.7%) than in the 68 countries study (42.7%) (2) and among seven Caribbean countries (54.3%), including in Dominica (43.1%) to 59.5% in Jamaica (59.5%) (4). In line with a previous investigation in seven Caribbean nations (4), the results of this study showed that the most prevalent external cause of injuries was fall-related injuries, and the three most common types of injuries were "fracture or dislocation", "cut or stab wound" and concussion.

Table 2. Associations with one or multiple injuries in the past 12 months

Variables	Unadjusted Odds Ratio (95% CI)	Adjusted Odds Ratio (95% CI)
Age in years ≤11-14 (32.8%) 15-16 (32.7%) 17-18 or more (34.5%)	1 (Reference) 0.88 (0.70, 1.11) 0.76 (0.62, 0.91)**	1 (Reference) 0.70 (0.55, 0.91)** 0.55 (0.43, 0.70)***
Gender Female (51.1%) Male (48.9%)	1 (Reference) 1.69 (1.44, 1.97)***	1 (Reference) 1.88 (1.53, 2.32)***
Parents provide necessities (81.7%)	0.70 (0.55, 0.90)**	1.15 (0.82, 1.60)
Experience hunger (3.8%)	1.83 (1.08, 3.10)*	1.01 (0.51, 2.01)
Current tobacco use (13.2%)	2.23 (1.76, 2.83)***	1.29 (0.96, 1.72)
Heavy alcohol use (19.0%)	1.85 (1.50, 2.28)***	1.69 (1.26, 2.26)***
Current cannabis use (5.7%)	2.87 (2.01, 4.08)***	1.65 (1.06, 2.56)*
Adequate physical activity (11.8%)	1.37 (1.07, 1.77)*	1.34 (1.01, 1.78)*
Physical education (3 or more days/week (32.6%)	1.15 (0.95, 1.39)	---
Truancy in the past month (26.6%)	1.46 (1.20, 1.78)***	1.23 (0.98, 1.56)
Psychological distress 0 (65.1%) 1 (20.5%) 2 or more (14.4%)	1 (Reference) 1.32 (1.08, 1.61)** 2.21 (1.67, 2.93)***	1 (Reference) 1.48 (1.16, 1.89)** 2.44 (1.73, 3.46)***
Peer support (mostly or always) (47.6%)	0.87 (0.72, 1.05)	---
Parental or guardian support Low: 0-1 (27.2%) Medium: 2 (26.7%) High: 3-4 (46.1%)	1 (Reference) 0.81 (0.64, 1.02) 0.68 (0.54, 0.85)***	1 (Reference) 0.94 (0.73, 1.21) 0.81 (0.63, 1.04)

CI = Confidence Interval; ***P< 0.001, **P< 0.01, *P< 0.05.

In agreement with previous studies (4,11-13), this study found that male sex and in unadjusted analysis poorer socioeconomic status (non-parental provision of necessities and the experience of hunger) were associated with annual injury. While this study did not find an association between peer and parental support and injury, a previous study (12) found an association between home environmental factors and injury. Parental support may have had a lessor significant influence in older than younger adolescents (14).

Consistent with previous studies (5,12,13,15), this investigation found a positive relationship between psychological distress, heavy alcohol use, current cannabis use and injury. It is possible that negative mood and the use of psychoactive substances increase the likelihood of injury behaviour (16). Therefore, it would be important to include mental health and substance use injury prevention programmes among adolescents (17). Moreover, this study found that daily participation in adequate physical activity was associated with a higher likelihood of injury. Higher frequency and intensity of participation in physical activity may increase the risk of injury (18).

Study limitations

The study was limited because of the cross-sectional design and only included school-going adolescents in Curaçao. The questionnaire used a self-report format, which has its limitations, in particular using a 12 months reference for injuries to occur. In addition, some data, including the place of injury, were not measured and should be included in future investigations.

CONCLUSION

Almost one in three of the participants had sustained at least one serious injury in the past 12 months and various factors (younger age, male sex, heavy alcohol use, current cannabis use, psychological distress, and physical activity) were found that could be targeted in programmes addressing injury prevention.

Appendix 1. Description of Variables and Response Options Analysed in This Paper

Variables	Question	Response options
Age	"How old are you?"	"11 years old or younger to 18 years old or older"
Sex	"What is your sex?"	"Male, Female"
Parents provide necessities	"During the past 30 days, how often did your parents or guardians provide for your necessities?"	"1= never to 5= always (coded 1–3=0 and 4–5=1)"
Hunger	"During the past 30 days, how often did you go hungry because there was not enough food in your home?"	"1=0 days to 7=All 30 days (coded 1=0 days, 2=rarely, and 3=sometimes/most of the time/always)"
Injury	"During the past 12 months, how many times were you seriously injured?" "(An injury is serious when it makes you miss at least one full day of usual activities (such as school, sports, or a job) or requires treatment by a doctor or nurse.)"	"1=0 times to 8=12 or more times (coded 1=0 and 2–8=1)"
Past month or current tobacco use	"During the past 30 days, on how many days did you smoke cigarettes/use any tobacco products other than cigarettes, such as such as *suruma*?"	"1=0 days to 7=All 30 days (coded 1=0 and 2-7=1)"
Heavy alcohol use (2 or more/day)	"During the past 30 days, on the days you drink alcohol, how many drinks did you usually drink per day?"	1 = Not drink in the past 30 days to 7 = 5 or more drinks (coded 1–3 = 0 and 4–7 = 1)
Current cannabis use	"During the past 30 days, how many times have you used marijuana (also called weed, pot, cannabis, ganja, or grass)?"	"1=0 days to 7=All 30 days (coded 1=0 and 2-7=1)"
Adequate physical activity	"Physical activity is any activity that increases your heart rate and makes you get out of breath some of the time. Physical activity can be done in sports, playing with friends, or walking to school. Some examples of physical activity are running, fast walking, biking, dancing, football, swimming, baseball, and cross-fit. During the past 7 days, on how many days were you physically active for a total of at least 60 minutes per day?"	"0=0 days to 7=7 days (coded 0-6=0 and 7=1)"
Physical education	"During this school year, on how many days did you go to physical education (PE) class each week?"	"1=0 days to 6=5 or more days (coded 1-3=0 and 4-6=1)"

Variables	Question	Response options
School truancy	"During the past 30 days, on how many days did you miss classes or school without permission?"	"1=0 days to 5= 10 or more days (coded 1=0 and 2–5=1)"
	Psychological distress	
No close friends	"How many close friends do you have?"	"1 = 0 to 4 = 3 or more (coded 1+=0, 0=1)"
Loneliness	"During the past 12 months, how often have you felt lonely?"	"1=never to 5=always (coded 1–3=0 and 4–5=1)"
Anxiety	"During the past 12 months, how often have you been so worried about something that you could not sleep at night?"	"1=never to 5=always (coded 1–3=0 and 4–5=1)"
Suicide ideation	"During the past 12 months, did you ever seriously consider attempting suicide?"	"Yes, No"
Suicide attempt	"During the past 12 months, how many times did you actually attempt suicide?"	"1=0 times to 5=6 or more times (coded 1=0 and 2–5=1)"
	Peer support	
Peer support	"During the past 30 days, how often were most of the students in your school kind and helpful?"	"1=never to 5=always (coded 1–3=0 and 4–5=1)"
	Parental or guardian support	
Parental supervision	"During the past 30 days, how often did your parents or guardians check to see if your homework was done?"	"1=never to 5=always (coded 1–3=0 and 4–5=1)"
Parental connectedness	"During the past 30 days, how often did your parents or guardians understand your problems and worries?"	"1=never to 5=always (coded 1–3=0 and 4–5=1)"
Parental bonding	"During the past 30 days, how often did your parents or guardians really know what you were doing with your free time?"	"1=never to 5=always (coded 1–3=0 and 4–5=1)"
Parental respect for privacy	"During the past 30 days, how often did your parents or guardians go through your things without your approval?"	"1=never to 5=always (coded 1–3=0 and 4–5=1)"

REFERENCES

[1] Sleet DA, Ballesteros MF, Borse NN. A review of unintentional injuries in adolescents. *Annu. Rev. Public Health* 2010;31:195–212.

[2] Han L, You D, Gao X, Duan S, Hu G, Wang H, et al. Unintentional injuries and violence among adolescents aged 12-15 years in 68 low-income and middle-income countries: A secondary analysis of data from the Global School-Based Student

Health Survey. *Lancet Child Adolesc. Health* 2019;3(9):616-26. doi: 10.1016/S2352-4642(19) 30195-6.

[3] Ricketts P, Bergeron M, Emmanuel R, Smith M. Trends in motor vehicle crash mortality in a small island developing state – the case of Dominica, 2000–2009. *Inj. Prev.* 2010;16:A243. doi:10.1136/ ip.2010.029215.866.

[4] Peltzer K, Pengpid S. Unintentional injury and social correlates among in-school adolescents in seven Caribbean countries. *MJSS* 2014;5(20): 2321-6. Doi:10.5901/mjss.2014.v5n20p2321.

[5] Peltzer K, Pengpid S. Unintentional injuries and psychosocial correlates among in-school adolescents in Malaysia. *Int. J. Environ. Res. Public Health2015*; 12(11): 14936-47. doi: 10.3390/ijerph12111 4936.

[6] World Health Organization (WHO). Global School-based Student Health Survey (GSHS). URL: http://www.who.int/chp/gshs/en/.

[7] Verstraeten S. The Curaçao Global School-based Student Health Survey (GSHS). Willemstad: Volksgezondheid Instituut Curaçao, 2015.

[8] World Health Organization (WHO) Global School-based Student Health Survey (GSHS). *2015 Curacao GSHS Questionnaire.* URL: https://www.who.int/ncds/surveillance/gshs/2015_GSHS_Curacao_Questionnaire.pdf.

[9] World Health Organization. *Physical activity fact sheet*, 2017. URL: http://www.who.int/mediacentre/factsheets/fs385/en/.

[10] Pengpid S, Peltzer K. Prevalence and correlates of behavioral non-communicable diseases risk factors among adolescents in the Seychelles: Results of a national school survey in 2015. *Int. J. Environ. Res. Public Health* 2019;16(15). pii: E2651. doi: 10.3390/ijerph16152651.

[11] Faelker T, Pickett W, Brison BJ. Socioeconomic differences in childhood injury: A population based epidemiologic study in Ontario, Canada. *Inj. Prev.* 2000;6:203–8.

[12] Mytton J, Towner E, Brussoni M, Gray S. Unintentional injuries in school-aged children and adolescents: lessons from a systematic review of cohort studies. *Inj. Prev.* 2009;15:111-24.

[13] Peltzer K. Injury and social determinants among in-school adolescents in six African countries. *Inj. Prev.* 2008;14:381-8.

[14] Wilson ML, Kamela BA, Dunlavy AC, Kigwangalla HA. Demoraphic and contextual influences in injury risk among adolescents in a low-income country setting: Results from a school-based survey in Tanzania. *Afr. Safety Promotion J.* 2012;10(2):41-9.

[15] Peltzer K, Pengpid S. Injury and social correlates among in-school adolescents in four Southeast Asian countries. *Int. J. Environ. Res.* Public Health 2012;9:2851-62.

[16] Pengpid S, Peltzer K. Unintentional injuries and socio-psychological correlates among school-going adolescents in four ASEAN countries. *Int. J. Gen. Med.* 2019;12:263-271. doi: 10.2147/ IJGM.S212350. *eCollection* 2019.

[17] Asbridge M, Azagba S, Langille DB, Rasic D. Elevated depressive symptoms and adolescent injury: examining associations by injury frequency, injury type, and gender. *BMC Public Health* 2014;14:190. doi: 10.1186/1471-2458-14-190.

[18] Räisänen AM, Parkkari J, Karhola L, Rimpelä A. Adolescent physical activity-related injuries in sports club, school sports and other leisure time physical activities. *Cogent. Medicine* 2016;3:1, DOI: 10.1080/2331205X.2016.1260786.

In: Adolescence in Curaçao
Editors: Soraya Verstraeten et al.
ISBN: 978-1-53617-522-6

Chapter 16

BEHAVIOURAL RISK FACTORS OF NON-COMMUNICABLE DISEASES AMONG SCHOOL-GOING ADOLESCENTS IN CURAÇAO: A CROSS-SECTIONAL NATIONAL STUDY

Supa Pengpid[1,2], DrPH and Karl Peltzer[*,2], PhD
[1]ASEAN Institute for Health Development, Mahidol University, Salaya, Phutthamonthon, Nakhon Pathom, Thailand
[2]Department of Research Administration and Development, University of Limpopo, Turfloop, South Africa

ABSTRACT

In this chapter we assess the prevalence and correlates of behavioural non-communicable diseases (NCD) risk factors among adolescents in

* ***Correspondence***: Professor Karl Peltzer, Department of Research Administration and Development, University of Limpopo, Turfloop Campus, Private Bag X1106, Sovenga 0727, South Africa. Email: kfpeltzer@gmail.com.

Curaçao. In the cross-sectional Curaçao "Global School-Based Student Health Survey (GSHS)" in 2015, 2,765 adolescents (median age 15 years) responded to questions on sociodemographic factors, substance use, psychological distress, protective factors and health risk behaviour. Six behavioural NCD risk factors (substance use, dietary behaviour, low physical activity and sedentary behaviour) were assessed by questionnaire in a classroom setting. Results indicate the prevalence of low physical activity was 88.2%, insufficient fruit and vegetable intake 83.5%, having soft drinks daily 60.9%, leisure-time sedentary behaviour 61.9%, current alcohol use 40.8% and current tobacco use 13.2%. From the six behavioural NCD risk factors, the mean was 3.5 (SD = 1.2), and 80.0% had at least three risk factors. In adjusted linear regression analysis, increasing age increased the odds and school attendance, living with both parents and high parental support decreased the odds for having multiple behavioural risk factors. A high co-occurrence of behavioural NCD risk factors was identified. Several risk factors (older age, sex, psychological distress, school truancy, living with no or a single parent, and poor parental support) for two or more individual and/or multiple behavioural NCD risk factors were identified that can be targeted in intervention programmes.

INTRODUCTION

"Non-communicable diseases (NCDs), including cardiovascular diseases, cancers, respiratory diseases, and diabetes, cause 71% of all deaths globally, and over 85% in low- and middle-income countries" [1]. Behavioural risk factors, such as "tobacco use, physical inactivity, the harmful use of alcohol and unhealthy diets all increase the risk of dying from a NCD."[1] "Caribbean countries, including Curaçao, are experiencing social, epidemiological, and demographic transitions shaped by the growing elderly population and the rise of NCDs-now responsible for 78% of all deaths"[2]. In the 2017 Curaçao national adult health survey, 64.9% were overweight or obese, 13.6% were smoking, 57.6% alcohol users, 18.8% were completely physically inactive, 16.1% had ≥ 2 fruits daily, 14.0% ≥ 2 vegetable servings daily, 28.5% consumed soft drinks daily, 40.8% ate food at least once a week from a fast food restaurant [3]. Evidence shows that behavioural risk factors are often acquired during the adolescence period and are then adopted in adulthood [4, 5]. There is a paucity of data on behavioural NCD risk variables in the adolescent population in Curaçao.

In a multi-country study (2003-2011) among adolescents, the prevalence of insufficient fruit and vegetable intake (FVI) was 74.3%, low physical activity 71.4%, alcohol use 15.7%, tobacco use 12.1%, and obesity 7.1% [6]. In the same study [6], the prevalence of having at least three NCD risk factors (of five risk factors) was 17.3% in the Americas, and 10.1% in Jamaica in 2010 and British Virgin Islands 22.9% in 2009 [6]. In a study among adolescents in Brazil, 58.5% reported being exposed to at least two of five behavioural risk factors at the same time [7], among adolescent in the Seychelles, 80.7% had 3-7 risk factors [8], and among adolescents in Nepal, 11.2% had 3-5 risk factors [9].

As reviewed in Pengpid and Peltzer [8], factors associated with individual and/or multiple behavioural NCD risk factors among adolescents, include male sex, older age, lower socioeconomic status, physical inactivity, insufficient physical activity, not attending physical education classes, overweight/obesity, psychological distress, school truancy and lack of peer and parental support. The study aimed to investigate the prevalence and correlates of behavioural NCD risk factors in adolescents in Curaçao.

OUR STUDY

Cross-sectional data from the 2015 Curaçao GSHS were analysed [10]. The study used a two-stage cluster sample design to produce data representative of all students enrolled in public secondary education, comparable to US Grades 1-6, in Curaçao. "At the first stage, 28 schools were selected with probability proportional to enrolment size, and at the second stage, 161 classes were randomly selected" [11]. All students in selected classes were eligible to participate after ethical approval in accordance with the *"WMA Declaration of Helsinki – Ethical Principles for Medical Research Involving Human Subjects"* and other permissions were granted and informed consent was obtained from parents and children; the overall response rate was 83% [11].

Table 1. Variable description

Variables	Question	Response options
Age	"How old are you?"	"11 years old or younger to 18 years old or older"
Sex	"What is your sex?"	"Male, Female"
Hunger	"During the past 30 days, how often did you go hungry because there was not enough food in your home?"	"1 = never to 5 = always (coded 1–3=0 and 4–5 = 1)"
	Behavioural risk factors	
Current tobacco use	"During the past 30 days, on how many days did you smoke cigarettes/use any tobacco products other than cigarettes, such as cigars, cigarillos, or electronic cigarettes?"	"1 = 0 days to 7 =All 30 days (coded 1 = 0 and 2-7 = 1)"
Current alcohol use	"During the past 30 days, on how many days did you have at least one drink containing alcohol?"	"1 = 0 days to 7 = All 30 days (coded 1=0 and 2-7 = 1)"
Fruits	"During the past 30 days, how many times per day did you usually eat fruit such as papaya, melon, banana, apples, grape, or pineapple?"	"1 = I did not eat fruit during the past 30 days to 7 = 5 or more times per day"
Vegetables	"During the past 30 days, how many times per day did you usually eat vegetables, such as carrots, beans, tomato, cabbage, or pumpkin?"	"I did not eat vegetables during the past 30 days to 7 = 5 or more times per day "
Soft drink consumption	"During the past 30 days, how many times per day did you usually drink carbonated soft drinks, such as Coke, Sprite, fria, monster, busta, RedBull, coco rico, and malta? (Do not include diet soft drinks.)"	1 = I did not drink carbonated soft drinks during the past 30 days to 7 = 5 or more times per day (coded 1=once or more/day)
Physical inactivity	"Physical activity is any activity that increases your heart rate and makes you get out of breath some of the time. Physical activity can be done in sports, playing with friends, or walking to school. Some examples of physical activity are running, fast walking, biking, dancing, football, swimming, baseball, and cross-fit. During the past 7 days, on how many days were you physically active for a total of at least 60 minutes per day?"	"0 = 0 days to 7 = 7 days (coded 0-6 = 1 and 7 = 0)"

Variables	Question	Response options
Leisure-time sedentary behavior	"How much time do you spend during a typical or usual day sitting and watching television, playing computer games, talking with friends, or doing other sitting activities, such as playing domino?"	"1 = Less than 1 hour per day… 3 = 3 to 4 hours per day …6 = 8 or more hours a day"
	Psychological distress	*"Yes, No"*
No close friends	"How many close friends do you have?"	"1 = 0 to 4 = 3 or more (coded 1+ = 0, 0 = 1)"
Loneliness	"During the past 12 months, how often have you felt lonely?"	"1 = never to 5 = always (coded 1–3 = 0 and 4–5 = 1)"
Anxiety	"During the past 12 months, how often have you been so worried about something that you could not sleep at night?"	"1 = never to 5 = always (coded 1–3 = 0 and 4–5 = 1)"
Suicide ideation	"During the past 12 months, did you ever seriously consider attempting suicide?"	"Yes, No"
Suicide attempt	"During the past 12 months, how many times did you actually attempt suicide?"	"1 = 0 times to 5 = 6 or more times (coded 1 = 0 and 2–5 = 1)"
	Protective factors	
School attendance	"During the past 30 days, on how many days did you miss classes or school without permission?"	"1 = 0 days to 5= 10 or more days (coded 1 =1 and 2–5 = 0)"
Physical education	"During this school year, on how many days did you go to physical education (PE) class each week?"	"1 = 0 days to 6 = 5 or more days (coded 1-4 = 0 and 5-6 = 1 two or more days)"
Peer support	"During the past 30 days, how often were most of the students in your school kind and helpful?"	"1 = never to 5 = always (coded 1–3 = 0 and 4–5 = 1)"
Religious person	"Do you think of yourself as a religious or spiritual person?"	"Yes, No"
Parents provide necessities	"During the past 30 days, how often did your parents or guardians provide for your necessities?"	"1 = never to 5=always (coded 1–3 = 0 and 4–5 = 1)"
Live with both parents	"Which adult family members do you live with?"	"1 = Both my mother and father to 5 = I do not live with any adult family members (coded 1 = 1 and 2-5 = 0)"
Parental supervision	"During the past 30 days, how often did your parents or guardians check to see if your homework was done?"	"1 = never to 5=always (coded 1–3 = 0 and 4–5 = 1)"

Table 1. (Continued)

Variables	Question	Response options
Protective factors		
Parental connectedness	"During the past 30 days, how often did your parents or guardians understand your problems and worries?"	"1 = never to 5 = always (coded 1–3 = 0 and 4–5 = 1)"
Parental bonding	"During the past 30 days, how often did your parents or guardians really know what you were doing with your free time?	"1 = never to 5 = always (coded 1–3 = 0 and 4–5 = 1)"
Parental respect for privacy	"During the past 30 days, how often did your parents or guardians go through your things without your approval?"	"1 = never to 5 = always (coded 1–3 = 0 and 4–5 = 1)"

MEASURES

The GSHS measure applied to this analysis was used in this survey (see table 1) [10]. "Inadequate FV consumption was classified as less than five or more servings in a day" [8, 12]. "Inadequate physical activity was defined as not daily at least 60 minutes of moderate to vigorous-intensity physical activity"[13]. "Sedentary behaviour was defined as spending three or more hours per day sitting"[14]. "The psychological distress items (no close friends, loneliness, anxiety, suicidal ideation and suicide attempt) were summed, and grouped into 0 = 0, 1 = 1 single and 2-5 = 2 multiple"[8]. "The four items on parental or guardian support were summed, and classified into three groups, 0-1 low, 2 medium and 3-4 high support" [8].

DATA ANALYSIS

Considering the complex design of the study, data analyses were conducted with "STATA software version 15.0 (Stata Corporation, College Station, TX, USA)." Descriptive statistics are used to provide frequencies, means and standard deviations. Multivariable logistic and linear regression analyses were utilized for assessing the associations between independent variables and individual and multiple behavioural risk factors. Data with missing information were excluded from the analyses. P values < 0.05% were considered significant.

FINDINGS

The sample consisted of 2,765 school students (median age 15 years, interquartile range 3 years), 51.1% females and 48.9% males, 3.8% had often experienced hunger, and 20.5% had a single and 14.4% multiple psychological distress. In terms of protective factors, 73.4% of students attended school in the 30 days, 32.6% had participated in ≥ 3 classes of physical education, 47.6% received frequently support by their peers, 69.0% considered themselves a religious or spiritual person, 81.7% were provided with necessities by their parents, 48.9% lived with both parents, and 72.8% had two to four parental support scores.

Regarding individual behavioural risk factors, 88.2% of students had low physical activity, 83.5% had insufficient FV intake, 60.9% consumed soft drinks daily, 61.9% engaged in leisure-time sedentary behaviour, 40.8% and 13.2% were currently using alcohol and tobacco, respectively. The total mean of the measured six behavioural NCD risk factors was 3.5 (SD = 1.2), and the distribution of the multiple occurrence of the behavioural risk factors was 0 = 0.4%, 1 = 3.2%, 2 = 16.4%, 3 = 31.1%, 4 = 29.3%, 5 = 15.5%, and 6 = 4.1%, and 80.0% had at least three risk factors (see table 2).

ASSOCIATIONS WITH INDIVIDUAL AND MULTIPLE BEHAVIOURAL RISK FACTORS

In the adjusted logistic regression model, being male was negatively associated with alcohol use and positively associated tobacco use. Older age increased the odds for alcohol use and inadequate FV intake. Multiple psychological distress was positively associated with alcohol and tobacco use. School attendance and high parental support were protective from both alcohol and tobacco use. Attending physical education classes was protective from inadequate FV intake. Having peer support was protective from soft drink consumption, and being a religious person was protective from both tobacco use and soft drink consumption. Living with both parents decreased the odds for alcohol use and soft drink consumption (see table 3).

Being male, having psychological distress and high parental support decreased the odds for inadequate physical activity. Older age, and the parental provision of necessities increased the odds for sedentary behaviour. Older age was positively and school attendance, living with both parents and high parental support were negatively associated with multiple behavioural risk factors (see table 4).

Discussion

Results found a significant co-occurrence of NCD behavioural risk factors (mean 3.5 and 80.0% had 3-6 risk factors). This result is higher than in a previous older investigation (17.3% 3-5 risk factors) in the Americas [6], Jamaica (10.1%) [6], and British Virgin Islands (22.9%) [6], but was similar to adolescents in the Seychelles (80.7%, 3-7 risk factors) (8). The prevalence of physical inactivity (< 7 days) (88.2%), insufficient FV intake (83.5%) and current alcohol use (40.8%) in this study was higher than in the older multi- low- and middle-income country study (71.4%, 74.3%, and 15.7% respectively), while current tobacco use (13.2%) in this study was similar to the global study (12.1%) [6]. In the 2017 Curaçao national adult health survey, also high rates of alcohol use (57.6%) were reported, while the intake of daily soft drinks (28.5%) was lower among adults than among adolescents in this survey (60.9%) [3].

Table 2. (Continued)

Variable	Sample	Current alcohol use	Current tobacco use	Inadequate fruit and vegetable consumption	Soft drink consumption	Inadequate physical activity	Leisure-time sedentary behaviour	Total behavioural risk factors
	N (%)	%	%	%	%	%	%	M (SD)
Parents provide necessities	2082 (81.7)	40.2	11.7	84.0	59.6	88.6	63.9	3.5 (1.2)
Live with both parents	1325 (48.9)_	35.7	12.1	83.2	57.4	89.1	61.1	3.4 (1.2)
Parental support								
0-1								
2	665 (27.2)	49.8	19.3	83.2	63.7	89.0	63.2	3.7 (1.2)
3-4	659 (26.7)	42.6	13.2	87.7	59.9	88.9	67.6	3.6 (1.1)
	1167 (46.1)	34.2	7.9	82.5	58.5	87.2	59.0	3.3 (1.2)

Table 2. Sample characteristics and distribution of behavioural risk factors of non-communicable diseases

Variable	Sample	Current alcohol use	Current tobacco use	Inadequate fruit and vegetable consumption	Soft drink consumptio n	Inadequat e physical activity	Leisure-time sedentary behaviour	Total behavioural risk factors
	N (%)	%	%	%	%	%	%	M (SD)
				Sociodemographics				
All	2765	40.8	13.2	83.5	60.9	88.2	61.9	3.5 (1.2)
Age (years)								
≤ 14	1054 (32.8)	22.7	10.1	80.4	61.5	88.0	54.5	3.1 (1.1)
15 or 16	828 (32.7)	43.8	14.5	84.5	63.6	88.7	64.1	3.6 (1.2)
≥ 17	877 (34.5)	54.5	14.9	85.7	57.6	88.0	66.6	3.7 (1.2)
Sex								
Female	1508 (51.1)	43.5	10.8	84.6	60.5	90.9	61.5	3.4 (1.2)
Male	1230 (48.9)	38.0	15.5	82.6	61.4	85.1	62.1	3.5 (1.2)
Hungry	102 (3.8)	38.8	24.5	79.2	69.8	89.1	60.7	3.7 (1.2)
Psychological distress	1719 (65.1)	37.1	10.1	85.2	58.1	88.8	60.4	3.4 (1.2)
0	531 (20.5)	42.2	14.2	83.6	64.1	85.6	65.8	3.6 (1.1)
1	379 (14.4)	54.4	20.7	81.0	66.9	87.8	65.7	3.7 (1.2)
2-5								
School attendance	1976 (73.4)	35.0	9.3	84.1	58.8	88.4	60.6	3.4 (1.1)
Attending physical education classes/ ≥ 3 week	826 (32.6)	43.2	14.8	80.1	60.8	86.3	63.6	3.5 (1.2)
Peer support	1241 (47.6)	40.5	11.7	85.2	56.5	86.8	64.7	3.5 (1.2)
Religious person	1717 (69.0)	40.0	10.4	83.5	61.9	87.6	62.3	3.5 (1.2)

Table 3. Associations with behavioural NCD risk factors (alcohol, tobacco, fruit and vegetable consumption, and soft drink consumption)

Variable	Current alcohol use	Current tobacco use	Inadequate fruit and vegetable consumption	Soft drink consumption
	AOR (95% CI)	AOR (95% CI)	AOR (95% CI)	AOR (95% CI)
		Sociodemographics		
Sex				
Female	1 (Reference)	1 (Reference)	1 (Reference)	1 (Reference)
Male	0.80 (0.66, 0.99)*	1.56 (1.11, 2.21)*	0.83 (0.64, 1.08)	1.00 (0.80, 1.25)
Age (years)				
≤14	1 (Reference)	1 (Reference)	1 (Reference)	1 (Reference)
15 or 16	2.31 (1.84, 2.91)***	1.50 (0.98, 2.29)	1.45 (1.11, 1.91)**	1.04 (0.78, 1.40)
≥17	3.62 (2.77, 4.72)***	1.35 (0.88, 2.07)	1.56 (1.15, 2.11)**	0.84 (0.62, 1.15)
Hungry	0.83 (0.49, 1.40)	1.32 (0.60, 2.89)	0.74 (0.40, 1.37)	1.16 (0.75, 1.52)
Psychological distress				
0	1 (Reference)	1 (Reference)	1 (Reference)	1 (Reference)
1	0.96 (0.70, 1.32)	1.12 (0.80, 1.55)	0.88 (0.69, 1.12)	1.18 (0.96, 1.45)
2-5	1.46 (1.08, 1.98)*	1.92 (1.17, 3.15)**	0.84 (0.62, 1.14)	1.32 (0.98, 1.78)
		Protective factors		
School attendance	0.54 (0.43, 0.68)***	0.47 (0.35, 0.63)***	1.03 (0.75, 1.42)	0.81 (0.62, 1.06)
Attending physical education classes/≥3week	1.20 (0.98, 1.46)	1.34 (0.98, 1.85)	0.72 (0.56, 0.92)**	0.97 (0.78, 1.22)
Peer support	1.09 (0.90, 1.33)	1.25 (0.94, 1.66)	1.12 (0.89, 1.42)	0.83 (0.69, 0.99)*
Religious person	0.88 (0.72, 1.08)	0.60 (0.47, 0.78)***	0.81 (0.63, 1.05)	1.34 (1.07, 1.67)*
Parents provide necessities	0.98 (0.73, 1.32)	1.10 (0.78, 1.55)	1.03 (0.75, 1.42)	0.81 (0.62, 1.06)
Live with both parents	0.77 (0.64, 0.93)**	0.92 (0.71. 1.19)	0.89 (0.68, 1.17)	0.76 (0.64, 0.91)**

Table 3. (Continued)

Variable	Current alcohol use	Current tobacco use	Inadequate fruit and vegetable consumption	Soft drink consumption
	AOR (95% CI)	AOR (95% CI)	AOR (95% CI)	AOR (95% CI)
Protective factors				
Parental support				
0-1	1 (Reference)	1 (Reference)	1 (Reference)	1 (Reference)
2	0.80 (0.62, 1.02)	0.75 (0.56, 1.01)	1.42 (0.97, 2.07)	0.94 (0.70, 1.27)
3-4	0.65 (0.50, 0.86)*	0.47 (0.33, 0.66)***	0.94 (0.71, 1.25)	0.93 (0.71, 1.23)

AOR = Adjusted Odds Ratio; CI = Confidence Interval; ***P< 0.001, **P< 0.01, *P< 0.05.

Consistent with previous findings [7, 9, 15], this investigation found that older age increased the likelihood of the co-occurrence of behavioural NCD risk factors in this adolescent population. Unlike findings from some previous investigations [16, 17], the results of this study found no association between not participating in physical education and multiple health risk behaviours. The findings of this study showed that having psychological distress increased the odds for alcohol and tobacco use, but decreased the odds for inadequate physical activity. It is possible that adolescents use alcohol and/or tobacco to cope with negative emotion or psychological distress [18]. This investigation found that school attendance, living with both parents, and higher parental support were protective from multiple behavioural NCD risk factors, which is consistent with findings of previous studies [19-21]. Interventions to reduce multiple behavioural NCD risk factors may want to reinforce attending school and promoting parental support among adolescents.

In agreement with previous studies [16, 17, 22], this study found that attendance of physical education was protective from inadequate FVI but not physical inactivity. Attendance of school was found protective from alcohol and tobacco use. It is possible that adolescents engage in substance use while absent from school. This finding supports the importance of

Table 4. Associations with behavioural NCD risk factors (physical inactivity, leisure-time sedentary behaviour, and total number of behavioural NCD risk factors)

Variable	Inadequate physical activity	Leisure-time sedentary behaviour	Total behavioural risk factors
	AOR (95% CI)	AOR (95% CI)	Adjusted Beta (95% CI)
Sociodemographics			
Sex			
Female	1 (Reference)	1 (Reference)	Reference
Male	0.49 (0.37, 0.67)***	1.06 (0.86, 1.30)	-0.09 (-0.21 to 0.04)
Age (years)			
≤ 14	1 (Reference)	1 (Reference)	Reference
15 or 16	1.15 (0.83, 1.60)	1.55 (1.20, 2.00)***	0.38 (0.24 to 0.52)***
≥ 17	1.04 (0.69, 1.56)	1.76 (1.42, 2.19)***	0.46 (0.31 to 0.62)***
Hungry	1.12 (0.54, 2.35)	1.03 (0.54, 1.94)	0.03 (-0.23 to 0.30)
Psychological distress			
0	1 (Reference)	1 (Reference)	Reference
1	0.64 (0.48, 0.85)**	1.14 (0.91, 1.43)	0.02 (-0.11 to 0.14)
2-5	0.67 (0.47, 0.95)*	1.23 (0.94, 1.60)	0.17 (-0.01 to 0.35)
Protective factors			
School attendance	0.86 (0.71, 1.10)	0.86 (0.71, 1.10)	-0.31 (-0.43 -0.20)***
Attending physical education classes/≥ 3 week	0.77 (0.58, 1.03)	1.02 (0.77, 1.35)	-0.02 (-0.14 to 0.09)
Peer support	0.78 (0.59, 1.04)	1.18 (0.99, 1.40)	0.02 (-0.09 to 0.13)
Religious person	0.80 (0.58, 1.10)	0.89 (0.72, 1.11)	-0.08 (-0.20 to 0.04)
Parent provide necessities	1.47 (0.97, 2.22)	1.41 (1.12, 1.76)**	0.12 (-0.13 to 0.26)
Live with both parents	0.92 (0.74, 1.14)	1.26 (0.95, 1.65)	-0.15 (-0.22 to -0.07)***
Parental support			
0-1	1 (Reference)	1 (Reference)	Reference
2	0.85 (0.56, 1.28)	1.13 (0.86, 1.49)	-0.06 (-0.19 to 0.08)
3-4	0.66 (0.44, 0.99)*	0.83 (0.61, 1.13)	-0.29 (-0.43 to -0.15)***

AOR = Adjusted Odds Ratio; CI = Confidence Interval; ***P< 0.001, **P< 0.01, *P< 0.05.

physical education and other school activities in promoting healthy behaviours. Parental support was protective from several behavioural NCD risk factors, including alcohol and tobacco use, and low physical activity. Peer support was found to be protective from soft drink consumption. Peer, parental support and school attendance can be utilized in programmes preventing substance use and improving dietary behaviour and physical activity.

REFERENCES

[1] World Health Organization (WHO). *Non-communicable diseases*, 2018. URL: https://www.who.int/news-room/fact-sheets/detail/non communicable-diseases

[2] Cho M, Marchand M, Vega E, Holder R, Luciani S, Constansia-Kook J, Moya J. Health systems strengthening for noncommunicable disease control and healthy aging: integrated actions in Aruba and Curaçao. *Rev. Panam. Salud. Publica.* 2019;43:e55. doi: 10.26633/ RPSP.2019.55. eCollection 2019.

[3] Verstraeten SPA, Griffith M, Pin R. The National Health Survey Curaçao 2017. Results, methods and tables. Volksgezondheid Instituut Curaçao (VIC) Martinus Centrum Curaçao Molenplein z/n, Otrobanda, 2017. [Dutch]

[4] McPherson KE, Kerr S, Morgan A, McGee E, Cheater FM, McLean J, Egan J. The association between family and community social capital and health riskbehaviours in young people: an integrative review. *BMC Public Health* 2013;13:971. doi: 10.1186/1471-2458-13-971.

[5] Selvan MS, Kurpad AV. Primary prevention: why focus on children & young adolescents? *Indian J. Med. Res.* 2004;120(6):511-8.

[6] Caleyachetty R, Echouffo-Tcheugui JB, Tait CA, Schilsky S, Forrester T, Kengne AP. Prevalence of behavioural risk factors for cardiovascular disease in adolescents in low-income and middle-income countries: an individual participant data meta-analysis. *Lancet Diabetes Endocrinol.* 2015;3(7):535-44. doi: 10.1016/S2213-8587(15)00076-5.

[7] da Silva Brito AL, Hardman CM, de Barros MV. Prevalence and factors associated with the co-occurrence of health risk behaviors in adolescents. *Rev. Paul. Pediatr.* 2015;33(4):423-30. doi: 10.1016/j. rpped.2015.02.002.

[8] Pengpid S, Peltzer K. Prevalence and correlates of behavioral non-communicable diseases risk factors among adolescents in the Seychelles: Results of a national school survey in 2015. *Int. J. Environ. Res. Public Health.* 2019;16(15). pii: E2651. doi: 10.3390/ijerph16152651.

[9] Dhungana RR, Bista B, Pandey AR, de Courten M. Prevalence, clustering and sociodemographic distributions of non-communicable disease risk factors in Nepalese adolescents: secondary analysis of a nationwide school survey. *BMJ Open* 2019;9(5):e028263. doi: 10.1136/bmjopen-2018-028263.

[10] World Health Organization (WHO). Global School-based Student Health Survey (GSHS). URL: http://www.who.int/chp/gshs/en/.

[11] Verstraeten S. The Curaçao Global School-based Student Health Survey (GSHS). Willemstad: Volksgezondheid Instituut Curaçao, 2015.

[12] World Health Organization (WHO) Diet, nutrition and the prevention of chronic diseases. Geneva, Switzerland: WHO, 2003.

[13] World Health Organization. Physical activity fact sheet, 2017. URL: http://www.who.int/mediacentre/factsheets/fs385/en/.

[14] Guthold R. Cowan MJ, Autenrieth CS, Kann L, Riley LM. Physical activity and sedentary behavior among schoolchildren: A 34-country comparison. *J. Pediatr.* 2010;157:43-9.

[15] Dumith SC, Muniz LC, Tassitano RM, Hallal PC, Menezes AM. Clustering of risk factors for chronic diseases among adolescents from Southern Brazil. *Prev. Med.* 2012;54(6):393-6. doi: 10.1016/j.ypmed.2012.03.014.

[16] Barbosa Filho VC, de Campos W, Bozza R, Lopes Ada S. The prevalence and correlates of behavioral risk factors for cardiovascular health among Southern Brazil adolescents: a cross-sectional study. *MC Pediatr.* 2012;12:130. doi: 10.1186/1471-2431-12-130.

[17] Tassitano RM, Barros MV, Tenório MC, Bezerra J, Florindo AA, Reis RS. Enrollment in physical education is associated with health-related behavior among high school students. *J. Sch.* Health 2010;80(3):126-33. doi: 10.1111/j.1746-1561.2009.00476.x.

[18] Chaplin TM, Niehaus C, Gonçalves SF. Stress reactivity and the developmental psychopathology of adolescent substance use. *Neurobiol. Stress.* 2018;9:133-9. doi: 10.1016/j.ynstr.2018.09.002. eCollection 2018 Nov.

[19] Allison MA, Attisha E. The link between school attendance and good health. *Pediatrics* 2019;143(2). pii: e20183648. doi: 10.1542/peds.2018-3648.

[20] Pengpid S, Peltzer K. Parental involvement and health risk behaviours among school-going adolescents in six African countries. *J. Psychol. Afr.* 2018; 28(3): 212-7. doi: 10.1080/14330237.2017. 1409481.

[21] Pengpid S, Peltzer K. Parental involvement, health behaviours and mental health among school-going adolescents in six Asian countries. ASR: *Chiang Mai. Univ. J. Soc. Sci. Hum.* 2016;3(2):115-32. https://doi.org/10.12982/CMUJASR.2016.0007.

[22] Silva DAS, Chaput JP, Tremblay MS. Participation frequency in physical education classes and physical activity and sitting time in Brazilian adolescents. *PLoS One* 2019;14(3):e0213785. doi: 10.1371/journal.pone.0213785. eCollection 2019.

SECTION TWO: ACKNOWLEDGMENTS

ISBN: 978-1-53617-522-6

Chapter 17

ABOUT THE EDITORS

Soraya Verstraeten, BAS, Msc, is the co-founder of the Institute of Public Health in Curaçao (Volksgezondheid Instituut Curaçao), where she coordinates data collection on health and healthcare through population-based surveys and data registration systems to support evidence-based policy making. As the principal investigator, she has led efforts on several large health studies, among which the national health surveys in 2013 and 2017 and the Global School-based Student Health Survey (GSHS) in 2015. Her main research interests are the determinants of good population health in a small island setting, which will culminate in the completion of her doctoral dissertation with the Erasmus MC in Rotterdam in April 2020. Email: S.verstraeten@vic.cw

Supa Pengpid, MPH, DrPH, MBA is a Professor at the ASEAN Institute for Health Development, Mahidol University Thailand since June 2013. She holds a Masterof Sciences in Public Health (MSc), Doctor of Public Health (DrPH in 2001) both from Mahidol University and Master of Business Administration (MBA in 2010) from Regenesys Business School, South Africa. She is a public health expert especially in health behaviour and public health. Her main research interests are health behaviour interventions in areas of chronic diseases prevention, obesity management, alcohol, HIV, TB and sexuality education, gender based violence and health systems research. Email: supaprom@yahoo.com

Karl Peltzer, MA Clin Psych, PhD, Dr Habil is a Research Associate in the Department of Research Administration and Development, University of Limpopo in South Africa. His research focuses on health promotion, risk behaviour and disease prevention, and socio-behavioural interventions on public health subject areas of alcohol, tobacco, cancer, tuberculosis and HIV control, nutrition, physical activity, hypertension, mental health, injury and violence prevention in low- and middle-income countries. Email: kfpeltzer@gmail.com

Joav Merrick, MD, MMedSci, DMSc, born and educated in Denmark is professor of pediatrics, Division of Pediatrics, Hadassah Hebrew University Medical Center, Mt Scopus Campus, Jerusalem, Israel and Kentucky Children's Hospital, University of Kentucky, Lexington, Kentucky United States and professor of public health at the Center for Healthy Development, School of Public Health, Georgia State University, Atlanta, United States, the former medical director of the Health Services, Division for Intellectual and Developmental Disabilities, Ministry of Social Affairs and Social Services, Jerusalem, the founder and director of the National Institute of Child Health and Human Development in Israel. Numerous publications in the field of pediatrics, child health and human development, rehabilitation, intellectual disability, disability, health, welfare, abuse, advocacy, quality of life and prevention. Received the Peter Sabroe Child Award for outstanding work on behalf of Danish Children in 1985 and the International LEGO-Prize ("The Children's Nobel Prize") for an extraordinary contribution towards improvement in child welfare and well-being in 1987. In 2017 appointed a Kentucky Colonel by the Commonwealth of Kentucky, the highest honor the governor can bestow to a person. Email: jmerrick@zahav.net.il

In: Adolescence in Curaçao
Editors: Soraya Verstraeten et al.
ISBN: 978-1-53617-522-6

Chapter 18

About the Institute of Public Health Curaçao (Volksgezondheid Instituut Curaçao)

The Institute of Public Health Curaçao (VIC) was established in July 2012 as an independent research institute of the Ministry of Health, Environment and Nature. VIC's purpose is to collect data on health and healthcare according to scientifically sound methods, with the main objective of informing the development and evaluation of health policies. To this end, VIC actively works together with other organizations in the public sector, with professional groups and their associations, and with international health organizations such as the PAHO/WHO, the CDC and RIVM. VIC currently has access to all kinds of up-to-date health information on population health in Curaçao from studies including national health surveys, health register and mortality data analyses, and national health accounts, and makes this information accessible through its website on www.vic.cw.

In: Adolescence in Curaçao
Editors: Soraya Verstraeten et al.
ISBN: 978-1-53617-522-6

Chapter 19

ABOUT THE ASEAN INSTITUTE FOR HEALTH DEVELOPMENT

The ASEAN Institute for Health Development (AIHD) was established in 1982 as the ASEAN Training Centre for Primary Health Care Development. It was a joint effort of Mahidol University, the Ministry of Public Health and the Department of Technical and Economic Cooperation (DTEC, now TICA) of the Royal Thai Government, with strong support from the Japan International Cooperation Agency (JICA).

AIHD is based on a forward-looking and conceptually challenging perspective on human resource development which aims to support the global strategy of "Health for all" through the primary health care approach advocated by the World Health Organization, an approach which is valid not only for Thailand but also other ASEAN countries.

AIHD has three key missions, namely education and training, technical services, and research and development, focusing on participatory community-based health and related program management, with a special emphasis on facilitating the paradigm shift from a "service-oriented" approach to a "development" approach in order to promote "Health for all" through human capacity building and community empowerment.

Vision

Center of excellence in research, education, professional services for innovative of sustainable health by 2020.

Mission

Provide transformative education for graduates to become leaders in health system management and sustainability. Enhance capacity related of public health workforce in relate to sustainable health development and develop innovative research for sustainable health.

Strategies

Excellence in research for health development models and sustainability. Transformative education. Innovative professional service for sustainable health and excellence in management for sustainable organization.

Website

www.aihd.mahidol.ac.th

In: Adolescence in Curaçao
Editors: Soraya Verstraeten et al.
ISBN: 978-1-53617-522-6

Chapter 20

About the Department of Research and Administration at University of Limpopo in South Africa

The Department of Research Administration and Development is a key Department at the University of Limpopo overseeing research performance across the university, developing and implementing policies aligned to the university's strategic plan (UL 2019 - 2023) goal 5, which is improving the university's research standing and status. The department further intends to accelerate professional, quality, efficient research output with the hope to generate funds for the university. Among its key research responsibilities, the department is responsible for managing and directing all aspects of planning, policy, performance, operational support for research and innovation activities and to implement technology transfer and intellectual property (IP) management strategy.

In: Adolescence in Curaçao
Editors: Soraya Verstraeten et al.
ISBN: 978-1-53617-522-6

Chapter 21

About the National Institute of Child Health and Human Development in Israel

The National Institute of Child Health and Human Development (NICHD) in Israel was established in 1998 as a virtual institute under the auspices of the Medical Director, Ministry of Social Affairs and Social Services in order to function as the research arm for the Office of the Medical Director. In 1998 the National Council for Child Health and Pediatrics, Ministry of Health and in 1999 the Director General and Deputy Director General of the Ministry of Health endorsed the establishment of the NICHD.

Mission

The mission of a National Institute for Child Health and Human Development in Israel is to provide an academic focal point for the scholarly interdisciplinary study of child life, health, public health, welfare, disability, rehabilitation, intellectual disability and related aspects of human development. This mission includes research, teaching, clinical work, information and public service activities in the field of child health and human development.

Service and academic activities

Over the years many activities became focused in the south of Israel due to collaboration with various professionals at the Faculty of Health Sciences (FOHS) at the Ben Gurion University of the Negev (BGU). Since 2000 an affiliation with the Zusman Child Development Center at the Pediatric Division of Soroka University Medical Center has resulted in collaboration around the establishment of the Down Syndrome Clinic at that center. In 2002 a full course on "Disability" was established at the Recanati School for Allied Professions in the Community, FOHS, BGU and in 2005 collaboration was started with the Primary Care Unit of the faculty and disability became part of the master of public health course on "Children and society". In the academic year 2005-2006 a one semester course on "Aging with disability" was started as part of the master of science program in gerontology in our collaboration with the Center for Multidisciplinary Research in Aging. In 2010 collaborations with the Division of Pediatrics, Hadassah Hebrew University Medical Center, Jerusalem, Israel around the National Down Syndrome Center and teaching students and residents about intellectual and developmental disabilities as part of their training at this campus.

Research activities

The affiliated staff have over the years published work from projects and research activities in this national and international collaboration. In the year 2000 the International Journal of Adolescent Medicine and Health and in 2005 the International Journal on Disability and Human Development of De Gruyter Publishing House (Berlin and New York) were affiliated with the National Institute of Child Health and Human Development. From

2008 also the International Journal of Child Health and Human Development (Nova Science, New York), the International Journal of Child and Adolescent Health (Nova Science) and the Journal of Pain Management (Nova Science) affiliated and from 2009 the International Public Health Journal (Nova Science) and Journal of Alternative Medicine Research (Nova Science). All peer-reviewed international journals.

National collaborations

Nationally the NICHD works in collaboration with the Faculty of Health Sciences, Ben Gurion University of the Negev; Department of Physical Therapy, Sackler School of Medicine, Tel Aviv University; Autism Center, Assaf HaRofeh Medical Center; National Rett and PKU Centers at Chaim Sheba Medical Center, Tel HaShomer; Department of Physiotherapy, Haifa University; Department of Education, Bar Ilan University, Ramat Gan, Faculty of Social Sciences and Health Sciences; College of Judea and Samaria in Ariel and in 2011 affiliation with Center for Pediatric Chronic Diseases and National Center for Down Syndrome, Department of Pediatrics, Hadassah Hebrew University Medical Center, Mount Scopus Campus, Jerusalem.

International collaborations

Internationally with the Department of Disability and Human Development, College of Applied Health Sciences, University of Illinois at Chicago; Strong Center for Developmental Disabilities, Golisano Children's Hospital at Strong, University of Rochester School of Medicine and Dentistry, New York; Centre on Intellectual Disabilities, University of Albany, New York; Centre for Chronic Disease Prevention and Control, Health Canada, Ottawa; Chandler Medical Center and Children’s Hospital, Kentucky Children’s Hospital, Section of Adolescent Medicine, University of Kentucky, Lexington; Chronic Disease Prevention and Control Research

Center, Baylor College of Medicine, Houston, Texas; Division of Neuroscience, Department of Psychiatry, Columbia University, New York; Institute for the Study of Disadvantage and Disability, Atlanta; Center for Autism and Related Disorders, Department Psychiatry, Children's Hospital Boston, Boston; Department of Pediatric and Adolescent Medicine, Western Michigan University Homer Stryker MD School of Medicine, Kalamazoo, Michigan, United States; Department of Paediatrics, Child Health and Adolescent Medicine, Children's Hospital at Westmead, Westmead, Australia; International Centre for the Study of Occupational and Mental Health, Düsseldorf, Germany; Centre for Advanced Studies in Nursing, Department of General Practice and Primary Care, University of Aberdeen, Aberdeen, United Kingdom; Quality of Life Research Center, Copenhagen, Denmark; Nordic School of Public Health, Gottenburg, Sweden, Scandinavian Institute of Quality of Working Life, Oslo, Norway; The Department of Applied Social Sciences (APSS) of The Hong Kong Polytechnic University Hong Kong.

Targets

Our focus is on research, international collaborations, clinical work, teaching and policy in health, disability and human development and to establish the NICHD as a permanent institute in Israel in order to conduct model research and policy.

Contact

Professor Joav Merrick, MD, MMedSci, DMSc
Director, National Institute of Child Health and Human Development, Jerusalem, Israel.
E-mail: jmerrick@zahav.net.il

SECTION THREE: INDEX

INDEX

C

D

I

J

K

L

M

N

O

P

R

S

T

U

V

W

Y